Building Your Otolaryngology Practice

Fiyin Sokoya

Building Your Otolaryngology Practice

A Playbook for Physician Success

Springer

Fiyin Sokoya
Wellstar Health Systems
Atlanta, GA, USA

ISBN 978-3-032-27396-3 ISBN 978-3-032-27397-0 (eBook)
https://doi.org/10.1007/978-3-032-27397-0

This Springer imprint is published by the registered company Springer Nature Switzerland AG
The registered company address is: Gewerbestrasse 11, 6330 Cham, Switzerland

Preface

When I was finishing training, I assumed that competence would be enough.

Like most surgeons, I believed that if I worked hard, took good care of patients, and did the right thing clinically, the rest would sort itself out. Practice would grow. Opportunities would appear. Fulfillment would follow.

Much of that turned out to be true. Some of it did not.

What I quickly realized, often the hard way, was that modern medical practice is shaped as much by systems, incentives, relationships, and timing as it is by skill. These forces are rarely discussed in residency or fellowship. When they are, they're often treated as peripheral, unseemly, or something you'll "figure out later."

Later is expensive.

This book exists because there is no coherent playbook for building a sustainable, high-impact career in otolaryngology. There are excellent textbooks on anatomy, pathology, and surgical technique. There is far less guidance on how to choose a practice model, how to build referrals without selling yourself, how to negotiate contracts intelligently, how to grow without burning out, or how to adapt as the landscape inevitably changes.

I did not write this book because I believe I have all the answers. I wrote it because I've had enough exposure to the questions—and enough scar tissue from learning them—to recognize patterns worth sharing.

Over the course of my career, I've trained and practiced within academic environments and large hospital systems, built a tertiary referral practice outside the ivory tower, and taken on leadership roles that forced me to understand the operational and financial realities behind clinical care. I've seen what works, what fails quietly, and what succeeds for reasons no one teaches.

More importantly, I've watched colleagues—smart, capable surgeons—struggle not because they lacked talent, but because they were navigating invisible rules with no map.

This book is not prescriptive. It does not argue that one practice model is superior to another, or that success looks the same for everyone. Instead, it aims to provide frameworks—ways of thinking about career decisions so that they are intentional rather than accidental.

To do that well, I knew my own perspective would not be enough.

Much of the insight in these pages comes from conversations with experienced otolaryngologists across the country: surgeons in academics, private practice, hospital-employed models, and hybrid arrangements; subspecialists and generalists; builders, leaders, and those who have chosen to stay deliberately small. Where they agree, I pay attention. Where they diverge, I explore why.

Their collective wisdom reinforces a simple truth: success in this field is rarely about being the smartest person in the room. It is about alignment—between your values and your environment, your skills and your incentives, your ambitions and your life outside medicine.

This book is written for residents, fellows, and early-career attendings—but it may be just as useful for those further along who feel successful on paper and unsettled in practice. If it helps you avoid a preventable mistake, reframe a decision, or define success on your own terms, it will have served its purpose.

Medicine is still a remarkable profession. Otolaryngology remains a uniquely diverse and rewarding specialty. But the path forward is no longer linear, and the default options are not always the best ones.

My hope is that this book helps you see the terrain more clearly—before you commit to a road that's difficult to leave. What follows is organized to move from the internal to the external—from self-knowledge to structure, from structure to strategy. The early chapters ask you to slow down and think before you act. The later chapters give you tools to act well: how to read a contract before you sign it, how to understand where your revenue actually goes, how to build a practice that doesn't require heroism to sustain, and how to negotiate from clarity rather than hope. If you are tempted to skip ahead to the tactics, I understand. But the physicians I interviewed who built the most durable careers all said some version of the same thing: the strategy only worked because the foundation was there first.

Atlanta, GA, USA Fiyin Sokoya

Introduction

A couple of years ago, a colleague called me on a Saturday morning to vent and share his cautionary tale. He was three years out of fellowship, hospital-employed, and by every external measure doing well. Good volume. Respected by peers. Patients liked him.

He wanted to leave.

The problem wasn't burnout in the way people usually mean it. He wasn't exhausted or disillusioned with medicine. He was disillusioned with his job—a job he had accepted quickly, negotiated poorly, and never fully understood until the daily reality set in.

His contract had seemed generous. The base salary was above the median. The signing bonus was meaningful. Relocation was covered. He had felt lucky.

What he hadn't examined closely enough was everything else. His wRVU threshold had been set using benchmarks that assumed a level of support he never received. His clinic template was designed for a predecessor with two APPs; he had half of one. Call was uncompensated but expected. And his non-compete—the clause he had barely read—covered a 40-mile radius in a metro area where 40 miles was effectively everywhere.

Now he wanted out, and the math was punishing. Tail coverage would cost him nearly $80,000, payable on departure. The non-compete meant starting over in a new city. His wife had just made partner at her firm. Their kids were in school. The cost of leaving had become so high that staying felt like the only option—even though staying meant producing at a pace that was slowly grinding him down inside a system whose incentives he now understood but could no longer change.

He wasn't a bad negotiator. He was a typical one. He had done what most physicians do: optimized for the number that felt most tangible—salary—and trusted that the rest would work itself out.

It didn't.

His story is not unusual. Versions of it surfaced in nearly every interview I conducted for this book. The details varied—academic politics, overhead surprises, private equity timelines, partnership terms that shifted after buy-in—but the underlying pattern was the same. A capable physician made consequential decisions without a framework for evaluating them, and discovered the cost only after the decisions had hardened into constraints.

This book is an attempt to provide that framework before you need it.

Most otolaryngologists leave training with a clear sense of *how* to practice medicine—but far less clarity about *where*, *with whom*, and *to what end*.

The traditional narrative suggests that careers unfold predictably: residency leads to fellowship or practice, early years are demanding but formative, and stability eventually follows. In reality, modern practice rarely adheres to a linear script. Instead, it is shaped by forces that are often invisible at the outset—financial incentives, institutional priorities, referral dynamics, geography, timing, and personal tolerance for risk and uncertainty.

These forces are not taught explicitly. They are learned piecemeal, through observation, trial and error, and—too often—through avoidable mistakes.

This book is not an argument against hard work, ambition, or excellence. It is an argument against drift.

Career drift is what happens when capable physicians move from opportunity to opportunity without a clear framework for evaluating tradeoffs. It is what leads some to feel trapped in roles they did not consciously choose, while others quietly build fulfilling practices that appear effortless from the outside. The difference is rarely talent. It is intentionality.

Otolaryngology is uniquely well positioned at the intersection of procedural medicine, longitudinal care, and subspecialization.

That diversity is a strength—but it also multiplies the number of viable career paths. Academic medicine, hospital employment, private practice, concierge models, and hybrid arrangements each offer distinct advantages and constraints. None is inherently superior. Each rewards certain values and penalizes others.

The problem is not that these models exist. The problem is that young physicians are often asked to choose among them before they have the language—or leverage—to understand what they are truly choosing.

This book is designed to supply that language.

Rather than prescribing a single path, it offers frameworks: ways of thinking about practice building that apply regardless of setting. It draws on the experiences of surgeons who have navigated different models successfully, identifying patterns that recur across geography, subspecialty, and career stage. Where there is consensus, it is highlighted. Where there is disagreement, the reasons for divergence are examined honestly.

Throughout, the emphasis is on alignment. Alignment between personal values and professional environments. Alignment between incentives and desired outcomes. Alignment between the work you do and the life you want to lead.

Practice building, in this sense, is not merely about growth. It is about design.

That design begins with self-knowledge.

Before considering contracts, compensation models, referral strategies, or productivity metrics, it is necessary to step back and ask a more fundamental question: *What are you actually trying to build?* A high-volume practice? A niche subspecialty? A leadership platform? Time flexibility? Financial independence? Academic influence? Geographic stability?

There is no universally correct answer—but there are answers that are more or less compatible with the choices that follow.

Chapter 1 begins there. Not with tactics, but with orientation. Not with the external landscape, but with the internal one. Because without clarity of direction, even the best opportunities can lead you somewhere you never intended to go.

The rest of the book builds outward from that foundation.

Acknowledgments

This book exists because of the generosity of others.

Every physician who agreed to be interviewed gave more than their time. They shared candor—about what worked, what didn't, and what they wished they had understood earlier. Many of the insights in these pages were not rehearsed or polished; they were offered honestly, often reflecting years of hard-earned perspective. That willingness to speak openly is rare, and it is the foundation of this book.

I am deeply grateful to Yadro Ducic, Andrew Winkler, Oswaldo Henriquez, Henry Barham, Jon Young, Ashley Agan, and David Parks for trusting me with their experiences and allowing their careers—both the successes and the inflection points—to be examined thoughtfully. Each of you has built a practice in a different way, but all of you share a commitment to rigor, integrity, and intentionality that continues to shape how I think about medicine and leadership.

I would also like to thank Kelley Young, AVP of Physician Relations at Wellstar. Her insight into practice building, physician engagement, and the often-overlooked mechanics of rounding, access, and relationship development within a health system added a critical operational perspective to this work. Understanding how practices grow from the institutional side—how trust is built, referrals are sustained, and alignment is created—helped round out the physician narratives with clarity and realism.

I am especially grateful to my wife, Courtnee. She has an uncanny ability to see what is possible long before I do, and she has consistently encouraged me to reach higher than I might have on my own. Writing this book meant long stretches of evenings and weekends spent in my office—time that could easily have been spent elsewhere. She understood that process without complaint and supported it with a generosity that made the work possible. Her perspective, patience, and belief in me have shaped this book in ways that may not be visible on the page but are present in every chapter.

Finally, I am grateful to the mentors, colleagues, trainees, and patients who were not formally interviewed but whose influence is embedded throughout these pages. Medicine is a collective endeavor. None of us build careers alone, and none of us see ourselves clearly without reflection from others.

If this book helps even one physician navigate their career with more clarity, agency, and alignment, it is because of the people acknowledged here.

Contents

1 **Charting Your Path** 1

2 **Understanding the Practice Landscape** 7

3 **Building Your Toolset** 17

4 **Financial Foundations** 23

5 **Productivity Optimization** 29

6 **Research and Innovation** 35

7 **Negotiating Contracts** 43

8 **Academic Practice** 51

9 **Hospital-Employed Practice** 61

10 **Private Practice** 69

11 **Concierge Medicine** 75

12 **Lessons from the Field** 85

13 **Adapting to the Future of Healthcare: Without Losing Yourself** 91

14 **Your Personalized Action Plan** 97

Index 103

1 Charting Your Path

The inscription at Delphi was not meant to inspire. It was meant to restrain.

Know thyself was a warning to those who believed that strength, intelligence, or ambition alone could protect them from error. The Greeks understood something modern professionals often forget: without clarity of purpose, capability becomes dangerous. Momentum replaces intention. Opportunity becomes a trap.

Medicine—and surgical training in particular—does not encourage self-knowledge. It rewards endurance. You advance by saying yes, by tolerating uncertainty, by moving forward before you feel ready. That conditioning serves you well in training. It serves you far less well when the structure disappears and you are asked to build a career instead of survive one.

Most otolaryngologists finish training highly skilled and deeply underprepared for that moment.

They know how to operate. They do not know how to orient.

From Motion to Direction

The first years out of training are dominated by motion. You are busy. You are learning. You are productive. These are good things—but they are not the same as direction.

F. Sokoya, *Building Your Otolaryngology Practice*,
https://doi.org/10.1007/978-3-032-27397-0_1

In *Nicomachean Ethics*, Aristotle distinguishes between action and purpose. Action, he argues, is meaningless without a telos—an end toward which it is directed. Without that end, activity becomes compulsive rather than constructive.

This is where many physicians get into trouble.

The earliest career decisions—first jobs, first contracts, first practice models—are often made under time pressure, with limited leverage, and minimal reflection. Offers are framed as rare opportunities. Declining feels risky. Pausing feels irresponsible. So decisions are made quickly, and rationalized later.

Oswaldo Henriquez described this arc plainly:

> When you come out of training, you're just happy to have a job. You've been asking 'pick me' your entire life. It takes five or ten years before you realize how much leverage you actually have.

The problem is not that early decisions are imperfect. The problem is that they are often made *without an explicit definition of where you are trying to go*.

Competence Is Assumed—Alignment Is Not

Greek philosophy placed enormous value on *arete*—excellence in function. A craftsman, a soldier, or a physician was expected to master his art. But mastery alone was never considered sufficient for a good life.

That distinction matters.

Every physician reading this book is competent. You would not have made it this far otherwise. Skill differentiates you from the general population, not from your peers. In practice, competence is assumed.

Henry Barham put it bluntly:

> Being able—the technical part—that's mostly done by the time you finish training. If you're not a good surgeon when you come out, you're probably not going to magically become one later.

And yet, many careers stall or sour not because the physician lacks skill, but because the environment they enter quietly rewards behaviors that conflict with their values.

Hospitals reward throughput. Academic centers reward visibility and grant capture. Private practices reward efficiency and local trust. None of these incentives are inherently wrong—but all of them shape behavior over time.

If you do not understand what a system rewards, you will eventually resent what it asks of you.

Success Is Not a Universal Metric

Aristotle's concept of *eudaimonia*—human flourishing—was never about wealth, status, or pleasure in isolation. It was about living in accordance with one's values over time. What constitutes flourishing varies by individual, but the requirement for alignment does not.

This is where most career dissatisfaction originates: optimizing for a definition of success that was never consciously chosen.

In training, success is externally defined. In practice, that definition fragments. Some physicians chase autonomy. Others seek stability. Some value growth, others predictability. Many want all of it—and are frustrated when trade-offs appear.

One senior surgeon reflected on how his definition of success changed:

> My kids don't care if I'm division chief or full professor. They care if I'm home. That changes how you define success.

This is not a sentimental observation. It is a structural one. When your personal definition of success diverges from the metrics your environment rewards, friction is inevitable.

The solution is not to reject ambition, but to define it more precisely.

There Is No "Right" Path

Plato warned against mistaking shadows for reality. In career building, prestige often functions as a shadow. It appears solid from a distance and collapses on contact.

There is no universally correct path in otolaryngology. Academic medicine, hospital employment, private practice, concierge models, and hybrid arrangements all produce fulfilled—and dissatisfied—physicians. What differs is not the label, but the fit.

The mistake is not choosing the "wrong" model. The mistake is choosing without understanding:

- What the model rewards
- What it constrains
- How it evolves over time
- Whether those constraints align with your values

As Seneca wrote, *"If one does not know to which port one is sailing, no wind is favorable."* In medicine, strong winds—high volume, good income, institutional support—can carry you very far in the wrong direction if you never chose a destination.

Careers Unfold in Phases

Life is cyclical, not linear. Modern careers are no different.

Early career rewards volume and flexibility. Mid-career rewards selectivity and leverage. Late career rewards optionality and perspective. Problems arise when physicians confuse a phase for an identity—when early-career tolerance becomes permanent self-betrayal, or when end-state goals are chased before foundations are built.

Intentional careers are marked by *periodic reflection*, not constant reinvention. A check-in every few years—asking whether your environment still serves your priorities—prevents dissatisfaction from becoming structural.

This is not instability. It is stewardship.

Values as Constraints

The Greeks did not treat virtue as aspiration, but as boundary. The *Golden Mean* was not about moderation for its own sake, but about sustainability.

Your values function the same way. They are not ideals to admire, but constraints to respect.

If autonomy matters deeply, certain environments will exhaust you.

If geographic stability is non-negotiable, some opportunities are incompatible.

If intellectual growth is essential, stagnation will corrode satisfaction regardless of compensation.

Ignoring these constraints does not make them disappear. It simply delays the cost.

From Philosophy to Practice

Self-knowledge does not make decisions easy. It makes them honest.

Once you know what you are trying to build, contracts become clearer. Practice models reveal their true costs. Comparison loses its grip. You stop chasing paths that look impressive and start choosing ones that are coherent.

The rest of this book moves outward—from internal clarity to external strategy. Financial structures, productivity, research, negotiation, and practice models all matter. But they are tools, not answers.

Without self-knowledge, tools create damage.

With it, they create leverage.

Before moving on, pause long enough to answer this question in writing:

What kind of life am I building—and what am I willing to trade to build it?

Everything that follows assumes you have begun to answer it.

The next chapter maps the terrain you'll be choosing from—not as it is described in recruiting brochures, but as it actually functions. Academic medicine, hospital employment, private practice, private equity, and the hybrid models that blur the lines between them. Each rewards certain values and quietly penalizes others. Understanding what you want is essential. Understanding what each system wants from you is what keeps that self-knowledge from being theoretical.

Understanding the Practice Landscape

2

Epictetus understood something that remains deeply relevant to physicians today: we are rarely harmed by circumstances alone. We are harmed by the stories we tell ourselves about those circumstances.

In medicine, those stories tend to be inherited. We absorb them during training—often consciously and sometimes unconsciously. Academic medicine is noble. Private practice is autonomous. Hospital employment is stable. Each label comes with assumptions that feel intuitive, almost timeless.

They are no longer reliable.

The landscape beneath those labels has shifted, quietly but decisively. If you don't update your mental model, you risk committing to a decades-long path based on a story that stopped being true years ago.

This chapter is about replacing myth with structure—so you can choose with clarity rather than momentum.

The Structural Shift: From Ownership to Employment

For most of modern medical history, physicians owned their practices. That ownership was not just financial—it conferred control over time, culture, and decision-making. In 2012, nearly 60% of

F. Sokoya, *Building Your Otolaryngology Practice*,
https://doi.org/10.1007/978-3-032-27397-0_2

US physicians practiced in physician-owned settings. By 2024, that figure had fallen to just over 42%, an 18-point drop in barely a decade [1].

During the same period, hospital ownership and direct hospital employment expanded steadily to the point that nearly half of all physicians now practice in hospital-affiliated environments [1].

This didn't happen because physicians suddenly decided they preferred employment. It happened because the business of medicine became more complex faster than most small practices could adapt. Reimbursement tightened. Payers consolidated. Staffing costs rose. Regulatory requirements multiplied. Electronic health records became mandatory—and expensive. Running a practice became a full-time job layered on top of clinical work [2].

Hospitals stepped into that gap because they could absorb risk at scale. They negotiated payer contracts, centralized administration, invested in infrastructure, and buffered volatility. The overhead costs are allocated and spread among hundreds of practices owned by the hospital system. For many physicians—especially early in their careers—employment became less a philosophical choice and more a practical response.

The mistake is not choosing employment. The mistake is assuming employment today looks like it did 20 years ago.

Academic Medicine: Mission, Metrics, and Reality

Academic medicine still attracts physicians for the right reasons: teaching, research, and exposure to complex pathology. But the internal mechanics of academic departments have changed in ways that trainees often underestimate.

Most academic ENT departments now rely heavily on clinical productivity, commonly measured in work Relative Value Unit (wRVU) and collections, to remain solvent [3]. Promotion criteria still emphasize scholarship and leadership, but daily expectations are often driven by access, throughput, and service-line economics.

What defines your lived experience in academia is not the mission statement. It's a handful of practical realities:

- Is protected time real, or theoretical?
- How aggressive are the wRVU expectations?
- Do you control OR block time, or compete for it?
- How heavy is the call burden?
- How are promotion and leadership decisions actually made?

One senior surgeon put it plainly:

> Academia still talks about mission, but the day-to-day runs on metrics. If you don't understand which ones matter, you'll feel that tension constantly.

The trap here is status bias**.** The label "academic" carries prestige and that prestige can mask a lack of control over schedule, staffing, and priorities. When an institution rewards visibility and output more than sustainability, physicians who value autonomy or balance often experience chronic friction.

Academic medicine can be deeply fulfilling—but only when the incentives match the ideals being advertised.

Hospital-Employed Practice: Platform or Cage

Hospital employment has grown because it solves real problems. Systems offer negotiated payer contracts, staffing infrastructure, marketing support, OR access, and integrated referral pathways. That scale matters.

By 2024, more than one-third of physicians practiced in hospital-owned groups, with another 12% directly employed or contracted by hospitals [1].

For otolaryngologists, hospital employment usually centers on service-line growth, access, and procedural throughput. Compensation is typically wRVU-based or heavily productivity-weighted, sometimes modified by quality or access metrics.

Whether this model works for you depends less on the contract than on the environment. The questions that matter are unglamorous but decisive:

- What is the *real* dollar-per-wRVU?
- Is call compensated—or just expected?
- Who controls your clinic template?
- How secure is your OR access?
- Are APPs extending your practice or replacing physician time?
- How much administrative reporting is required?

One physician described the difference succinctly:

> In the right system, employment is leverage. In the wrong one, it's just pressure with a paycheck.

That distinction rarely shows up in the offer letter. It reveals itself over time.

The Masked Model: Hospital Employment Wearing Academic Clothing

One of the most consequential—and least openly discussed—models today is hospital employment presented as academic medicine.

Systems such as Banner University, Wellstar/MCG, and similar university-affiliated networks offer faculty titles, trainees, and academic branding. On the surface, these environments look indistinguishable from traditional academic departments.

Structurally, many function much closer to hospital-employed practices.

Productivity-driven compensation is common. Research time is often limited or selectively funded. Governance frequently resides with the hospital rather than the university. Marketing emphasizes the institution, not individual physicians.

For some surgeons, this hybrid model is ideal: complex cases, teaching opportunities, and system resources without the grant-driven pressure of classic academia. For others, it creates dissonance—academic expectations layered on top of employed constraints.

As one interviewee warned:

> The danger isn't the model. The danger is thinking you're joining one thing and realizing later you joined something else.

In these environments, titles matter far less than answers to basic questions: Who controls your time? How is success measured? Where does decision-making authority actually sit?

Private Practice: Autonomy, Compounding, and the Price of Ownership

Private practice is often talked about in absolutes—either as the last refuge of physician autonomy or as a dying relic crushed by modern healthcare economics. Neither framing is particularly useful.

The truth is simpler and more uncomfortable: private practice is not freedom from constraint. It is ownership of constraint.

When you own a practice, you own everything that comes with it—culture, staffing, overhead, payer relationships, scheduling, and reputation. That ownership cuts both ways. It gives you real control over how you practice medicine, but it also exposes you directly to the pressures of the system.

Henry Barham put it plainly:

> Private practice isn't about doing whatever you want. It's about deciding which problems you're willing to own.

That distinction matters. In private practice, autonomy is real—but so is accountability. If access is poor, that's your problem. If staffing is unstable, that's your problem. If payer mix deteriorates, that's your problem. The upside is that when things go well, the compounding effects accrue to you, not to an institution.

The metrics that actually determine whether a private practice thrives are not abstract. They are concrete and operational:

- Overhead as a percentage of collections
- Payer mix and negotiated rates
- New-patient access and referral conversion
- Scheduling lead times
- Performance of ancillaries such as audiology, allergy, or in-office procedures

Physicians who succeed in private practice tend to understand this early. They treat reputation as an asset that compounds over time, not as something to be marketed aggressively.

That compounding—of trust, reliability, and local reputation—is something large systems struggle to replicate. It's also why many private practices remain viable even as consolidation accelerates.

At the same time, it's important not to romanticize the model. Private practice today exists in a more hostile environment than it did 20 years ago. Payer pressure is real. Administrative burden is real. Staffing volatility is real. This is why many successful groups now adopt hybrid structures—professional services agreements, management services, or hospital partnerships—to offload selected risks while preserving governance.

Private practice still works. But it works best for physicians who understand that autonomy and risk are inseparable, and who are intentional about which risks they are willing to carry.

Private Equity: Liquidity, Leverage, and the Cost of Time

Private equity enters the physician conversation carrying a lot of emotional weight. For some, it represents betrayal of the profession. For others, it looks like financial salvation. Both reactions miss the point.

Private equity is not a philosophy. It is a financial instrument.

At its core, private equity does three things well: it consolidates fragmented markets, standardizes operations, and creates liquidity. That liquidity can be enormously attractive—particularly to late-career physicians who have built valuable practices but lack a clean exit.

Dr. Ducic explained:

> Private equity makes a lot of sense when you're five or ten years from being done. It's a terrible deal if you're just getting started.

That framing is critical.

Private equity firms operate on defined timelines, typically aiming to exit investments within 3 to 8 years [4]. Growth is driven by scale, margin expansion, and operational efficiency. In practice, that often means higher productivity expectations, tighter controls, and increased use of non-physician providers.

For early-career physicians, the implications are subtle but important. You are stepping into a system whose primary obligation is not to patients, or even to physicians, but to investors. That doesn't make the care bad—but it does change priorities.

David Parks captured the trade-off succinctly:

> You're not really joining a practice. You're joining a business plan.

This is why private equity often works best as an exit strategy, not an entry point. For established physicians, it can convert years of effort into immediate liquidity while allowing continued clinical work for a defined period. For younger physicians, it can limit autonomy precisely at the stage when learning, experimentation, and flexibility matter most.

This is not a moral argument against private equity. It's a structural one. Private equity changes who the practice ultimately serves—and on what timeline.

The mistake is not partnering with private equity. The mistake is doing so without understanding where you sit in that lifecycle, and how much control you are willing to trade for certainty.

Incentives Shape Identity

There is a reason so many physicians describe burnout not as exhaustion, but as *misalignment*. Psychology has a name for this: behavioral shaping through incentives. Over time, people do not simply work within systems—they adapt to them. What is measured becomes what matters. What is rewarded becomes what is repeated. What is tolerated becomes normalized.

This is not a moral failing. It is human nature.

In behavioral psychology, this is called *operant conditioning*. In organizational psychology, it's framed as *incentive alignment*. In Stoic philosophy, it was understood more simply: if you place yourself in an environment that pulls you in a direction you do not wish to go, eventually you will drift there anyway.

That is why the practice landscape matters so much.

If you practice in a system that rewards speed over depth, you will become faster—whether or not that aligns with how you want to practice. If you work in an environment that values visibility over sustainability, you will feel pressure to perform rather than to endure. If you choose a model that prioritizes liquidity over longevity, your decisions will be shaped by timelines that are not your own.

None of this happens overnight. It happens quietly, incrementally, and almost invisibly.

The goal of this chapter is not to persuade you toward a particular model. It is to make you aware of a deeper truth: your environment will shape you far more than your intentions will. Motivation fades. Values erode under constant friction. Structure, on the other hand, is relentless.

Epictetus warned that we are not disturbed by things themselves, but by our judgments about them. In medicine, one of the most dangerous judgments is believing that a system will bend to your values simply because you hold them strongly enough.

It won't.

The work, then, is not to find the perfect practice model. It is to place yourself in a structure whose incentives pull you in roughly the same direction you already want to go. When that happens, discipline feels lighter, burnout is less likely, and success becomes more sustainable.

The next chapters move away from structure and toward agency—what you can control regardless of where you practice. But that control only works once you've chosen terrain that doesn't quietly work against you. Choosing the right terrain is necessary. It is not sufficient. The next chapter turns to the behaviors that compound regardless of setting—the habits of communication, availability, and institutional awareness that separate physicians who feel trapped from those who quietly accumulate options. These are not glamorous skills. They are the ones that, years later, determine whether you have leverage or merely a title.

Bibliography

1. American Medical Association. Physician practice benchmark survey 2024. AMA; 2024.
2. Kane CK. Policy research perspectives: updated data on physician practice ownership. AMA; 2024.
3. Association of American Medical Colleges. Faculty salary and productivity report. AAMC; 2023.
4. Borsa J, et al. Private equity investment in physician practices: trends and implications. Health Affairs Scholar; 2024.

Building Your Toolset 3

By the time you reach this point in the book, one reality should be clear: you do not control the healthcare system.

You don't control payer consolidation, hospital governance, or private equity timelines. You may not even control the practice model you enter early in your career.

That realization can feel unsettling—or it can feel clarifying.

This chapter is about what remains firmly within your control.

Across every interview I conducted—academic surgeons, private practitioners, hospital-employed physicians, and hybrid leaders—a consistent pattern emerged. Durable, satisfying careers were not built by finding the perfect system. They were built by mastering a small set of behaviors that compound quietly over time.

That set of behaviors is your toolset.

From Structure to Agency

The Stoics made a sharp distinction between what is *up to us* and what is not. Anxiety, they argued, comes from confusing the two. Freedom comes from focusing your effort where it actually matters.

The same principle applies to practice building.

F. Sokoya, *Building Your Otolaryngology Practice*,
https://doi.org/10.1007/978-3-032-27397-0_3

Once you understand the structure you're operating within, the question becomes practical: *How do I operate inside imperfect systems without being consumed by them?*

The answer is not a clever strategy or a shortcut. It's a series of habits—often unglamorous—that shape reputation, referrals, leverage, and optionality.

As Dr. Barham put it bluntly:

> Nobody remembers your mission statement. They remember whether you picked up the phone.

That is where agency begins.

Time Is the First Currency

Early in practice, time is mispriced.

You are busy, but you are also unusually flexible. Your clinic templates aren't saturated. Your referral streams are still forming. You have energy—and margin—that will not exist forever.

Experienced physicians recognize this for what it is: an investment window.

Dr. Oswaldo Henriquez, reflecting on his transition years, described it this way:

> The first year or two is when you actually have time to do things outside the OR. If you don't use that time to build relationships, you're going to feel it later.

This isn't about working more hours. It's about deploying time deliberately—rounding, meeting referring physicians, giving talks, joining committees, and learning how your system actually functions.

Time spent building trust early reduces friction later. Time spent avoiding that work compounds regret.

Reputation Is Behavioral, Not Promotional

One of the most common misconceptions among early-career physicians is that reputation is something you market.

It isn't.

Reputation is the sum of how you behave when no one is watching. How you respond to inconvenience. How you communicate when there is nothing obvious to gain. How predictable you are under ordinary circumstances.

Dr. Ducic, who has built a referral base that spans decades, described his approach simply:

> I never went out asking for referrals. I just took care of the patient, communicated clearly, and made life easier for the referring doctor. Over time, that compounds.

That compounding effect is slow—but powerful. It's also fragile. One dismissive interaction can undo months of goodwill.

The strongest reputations are quiet. They spread laterally, not loudly.

Communication Is a Force Multiplier

If there is one underappreciated skill in modern practice building, it is communication.

Electronic medical records were meant to improve information flow. In many cases, they've done the opposite. Notes are longer, less readable, and less personal. Referring physicians are often left out of the loop.

The physicians who stand out do something deceptively simple: they close the loop.

They call. They dictate concise letters. They explain plans clearly. They respect the cognitive load of the referring provider.

Dr. David Parks, reflecting on decades of practice, emphasized this repeatedly:

> People don't refer because you're smart. They refer because you're reliable and easy to work with.

Reliability, it turns out, is a communication skill.

The Three A's—Revisited

Across interviews, the same framework surfaced again and again: *Able, Available, Affable*.

What experience clarifies is their hierarchy.

Technical ability is assumed. You wouldn't be here otherwise. It differentiates you from the general public, not from your peers.

Availability, on the other hand, is rare—and memorable. Picking up the phone. Squeezing in a patient. Responding promptly. Availability is the best ability.

Affability is the multiplier.

Dr. Jon Young, who has built subspecialty programs inside large systems, put it plainly:

> You can be great technically, but if you're a pain to deal with, people will route around you.

This isn't about being agreeable. It's about being professional, respectful, and predictable. The best ability is availability.

Social Media: Amplifier, Not Foundation

Social media deserves a sober assessment.

For some physicians, it accelerates awareness. It signals expertise to peers. It helps patients understand what you do. For others, it's a distraction.

The mistake is believing social media creates trust.

It doesn't.

As Dr. Henriquez noted:

> It helps people know what you do. It doesn't make them trust you.

Social media amplifies what already exists. If your fundamentals are strong—outcomes, communication, availability—it can magnify them. If they're weak, it magnifies that too.

Trust is earned offline.

Social media also helps bridge the familiarity gap between patients and physicians.

Dr. Agan noted: "Social media doesn't create trust—but it helps people find you. Patients will binge your content, and by the time they meet you, they feel like they already know you."

Committees, Leadership, and the Long Game

To early-career physicians, committees often feel like a waste of time. Meetings feel inefficient. Leadership feels abstract.

Experienced physicians see them differently.

Committees are where decisions get made. They're where relationships form across departments. They're where informal influence accumulates.

Dr. Parks captured the reality succinctly:

> If you don't have a seat at the table, you're probably on the menu.

You don't need to join every committee. You do need to understand how your institution works—and who actually holds power.

That knowledge pays dividends later, when you need OR time, staffing support, program development, or protection during periods of change.

Metrics That Actually Matter

Every system tracks metrics. Not all of them matter equally to you.

Early in practice, the most useful metrics are not national percentiles or abstract benchmarks. They are local and directional:

- New patient volume over time
- Stability of referral sources
- Clinic access and lead times
- OR utilization and block efficiency
- wRVU trajectory relative to effort

Metrics aren't about ego. They're feedback. Used correctly, they reveal leverage points before frustration sets in.

Optionality Is the Goal

The purpose of this toolset is not growth for its own sake.

It is optionality.

Optionality is the ability to say no. To renegotiate. To change direction. To walk away if necessary.

Physicians with strong reputations, stable referral streams, and institutional credibility have options. Those who neglect these fundamentals often feel trapped—not because they lack skill, but because they delayed investing in leverage.

Dr. Barham reflected on this later in his career:

> The best feeling wasn't the money. It was realizing I didn't have to take the next offer.

That freedom is built quietly, over time.

The Quiet Work That Compounds

None of the tools in this chapter are glamorous. They won't go viral. They don't generate immediate reward.

But they compound.

Into trust. Into referrals. Into credibility. Into leverage. Into the ability to shape your practice rather than be shaped by it.

In the next chapter, we'll turn to the financial foundations of practice building—not as an end, but as infrastructure. Because money, like reputation and structure, is most powerful when it supports what you're trying to build rather than dictating it.

4 Financial Foundations

I didn't truly understand healthcare finance until embarrassingly late.

Like most physicians, I thought I had a reasonable grasp of money. I knew my salary. I understood wRVUs in the abstract. I could read a paycheck and manage my personal expenses. I assumed that was enough.

It wasn't.

The real shift came during my MBA program, when I was forced to read healthcare financial statements the way executives and investors do. Around that time, I opened HCA's annual financial report—not a summary or a blog post, but the actual document. What stood out immediately were not the clinical buzzwords, but the hard realities: operating margins, payer mix, service-line contribution, capital allocation, debt structure, and downstream revenue capture.

Suddenly, the things I had experienced intuitively as a clinician made sense. The obsession with access. The pressure around OR utilization. The relentless focus on throughput. These weren't arbitrary administrative behaviors. They were financial imperatives.

That was the moment I realized something uncomfortable: I had been making career decisions inside a system whose economics I did not understand.

This chapter exists to shorten that learning curve.

F. Sokoya, *Building Your Otolaryngology Practice*,
https://doi.org/10.1007/978-3-032-27397-0_4

Why Financial Literacy Is No Longer Optional

There was a time when you could be clinically excellent, financially naïve, and still end up fine. That era is fading.

Healthcare has consolidated rapidly, margins have tightened, and risk has shifted. Small inefficiencies that once disappeared into the noise are now exposed. Physicians who do not understand the financial mechanics of their environment are increasingly vulnerable, regardless of practice model.

This is not conjecture. A systematic review of financial literacy among healthcare professionals found that the majority of physicians and trainees lack formal education in personal and professional finance, with studies showing that up to 80% of residents receive no financial planning education during training. Even more concerning, 92% of surgical program directors reported that residents lacked the skills to manage their finances effectively [1]. Separate studies have linked this financial illiteracy to higher rates of stress, burnout, and delayed career satisfaction [2].

In other words, financial literacy is no longer a "nice to have." It is a core professional competency.

This does not mean you need to become a finance expert. It means you need to understand enough to recognize when incentives are misaligned—and when the system is quietly shifting risk onto you.

A Quick Reality Check

If you can't answer these questions confidently, you are under-informed for modern practice:

- Do you know how your hospital or practice actually makes money?
- Do you know which service lines subsidize others?
- Do you know your true dollar-per-wRVU—not the advertised rate?

- Do you know where the revenue you personally generate actually goes?
- Do you know which costs scale with volume and which don't?

This isn't trivia. These answers shape your autonomy.

Two Financial Realities You Must Hold at the Same Time

Physicians often oscillate between two extremes. Some ignore money entirely, trusting that "medicine will take care of me." Others become consumed by it, allowing income to dictate every decision. Both approaches are incomplete.

Your personal finances create optionality. A strong balance sheet gives you the ability to negotiate without fear, leave unhealthy environments, and absorb short-term volatility without panic. As Dr. Jon Young put it during our conversation, *"Live below your means. Get out of debt. Once you do that, you're in a completely different mindset."* Debt narrows choices. Liquidity widens them.

At the same time, practice economics shape your daily life. Whether you are employed, academic, hybrid, or private, you are participating in an economic system. Ignoring that reality does not insulate you from it—it simply makes you reactive inside it.

This is where many physicians get hurt: they optimize clinically inside systems they do not economically understand.

Revenue: What Actually Pays You (And What Doesn't)

Most physician income ultimately flows through a mix of base salary, productivity incentives, quality or access bonuses, call pay, ancillary services, and downstream value. The mistake is assuming all of these are equally within your control.

Nowhere is this misunderstanding more common than with wRVUs.

wRVUs and Collections

wRVUs were never designed as a compensation tool; they were created to standardize Medicare payment for physician work. Over time, they became the dominant currency of employed medicine, including in academic settings [3].

Once you are paid on wRVUs, your workday changes in subtle but important ways. Clinic templates tighten. Documentation time increases without direct compensation. Access and throughput begin to outweigh complexity. Support staff—scribes, APPs, coordinators—become the hidden variable that determines whether productivity expectations feel reasonable or crushing.

This is why two physicians with identical wRVU targets can have radically different experiences. The difference is not work ethic; it is resourcing. If you don't understand how wRVUs interact with staffing and support, you may assume you are inefficient when you are simply under-resourced.

Collections tell a different story. While collections matter most in private and hybrid models, they matter everywhere. They reveal payer mix, contract strength, and the true economic value of your work—whether or not you ever see that money directly. Collections explain why hospitals tolerate loss-leading clinics while fiercely protecting procedural service lines.

Cash Pay and Aesthetics: Knowing Which Levers You Control

One of the clearest explanations of cash-pay economics came from *Dr. Andrew Winkler*, an academic facial plastic surgeon who has built a robust aesthetic practice inside a university system.

His insight was deceptively simple: *"You can charge your surgeon's fee whatever you want. What you don't control is the facility or anesthesia."*

That distinction clarifies where pricing power actually lives. It also explains why so many surgeons misjudge their leverage in cash-pay work.

Winkler also described a pattern familiar to many early-career surgeons: *"When I first started out, I discounted a lot. As I've gotten busier, I don't discount very much at all."* Discounting is often a phase driven by uncertainty. As demand becomes real, pricing stabilizes.

He reframed so-called low-value services in a way that is both honest and strategic: *"Botox is such a commodity… I'm doing it to get people in the door."* Commodities attract attention. Premium work sustains practices.

Cash pay economics also lead to pricing transparency and could increase patient trust in the system.

Dr. Agan surmised: Once patients understand the real costs—facility, anesthesia, everything—they realize the surgeon's fee isn't the biggest piece. When the pricing is transparent, trust comes much easier.

Overhead: The Variable That Decides Everything

If revenue is what people talk about, overhead is what determines survival.

In private practice, overhead dictates whether growth produces wealth or exhaustion. In employed practice, overhead still exists—it is simply hidden. It determines how much support you receive, how many staff you are allocated, and how hard you must work to justify additional resources.

This is why so many physician-owned practices have sold over the past decade. Rising administrative and operational costs outpaced what many groups could absorb [2].

As Dr. Henry Barham summarized it succinctly, *"Overhead matters more than revenue."* That truth becomes obvious only after you've lived through it.

Private Equity: Understanding the Clock

Private equity is neither savior nor villain. It is a structure—and it runs on a timeline.

A 2024 analysis in *Health Affairs Scholar* found that among hundreds of physician practice acquisitions, more than half exited within 3 years, and nearly all were sold to another private equity firm rather than back to physicians [4]. That timeline matters.

For late-career physicians, private equity can convert years of work into immediate liquidity. For early-career physicians, it often introduces misaligned incentives at precisely the stage when learning, experimentation, and autonomy matter most.

You are not just joining a practice. You are joining a deal cycle.

A Practical Definition of Financial Success

Financial success is not about maximizing income. It is about building insulation.

Insulation looks like liquidity that absorbs life events without panic, margin that buys time and support, understanding that enables negotiation, and optionality that allows you to leave unhealthy environments.

Money is most powerful when it removes fear from decision-making. That is its role in practice building.

Bibliography

1. Sherrill WC, et al. Financial literacy among healthcare providers: a systematic review. 2024.
2. Kane CK. Policy research perspectives: updated data on physician practice ownership. American Medical Association; 2024.
3. Association of American Medical Colleges. Faculty salary and productivity report. AAMC; 2023–2025.
4. Singh Y, et al. Life cycle of private equity investments in physician practices. Health Affairs Scholar; 2024.

Productivity Optimization

5

By the time most physicians reach independent practice, effort is no longer the limiting factor.

You already know how to work hard. You have tolerated long hours, high cognitive load, emotional stress, and physical fatigue. Productivity problems that arise later are rarely about discipline or motivation. They are about where time goes—and why so much of it leaks out of the system.

This chapter is about reclaiming that lost time.

Not by working longer days, but by understanding how productivity is actually created—and destroyed—in modern practice.

Time Is the Irreducible Constraint

Money matters. Metrics matter. But time is the one resource that cannot be manufactured.

Every practice model ultimately allocates time: clinic slots, OR blocks, administrative hours, call responsibilities. How that time is structured determines how productive you are, how much energy you have left at the end of the day, and how sustainable your career becomes.

The common mistake is trying to increase output without stabilizing the container. Physicians add clinic sessions, squeeze in cases, or work later into the evening. Output may rise temporarily, but the cost is deferred—and cumulative.

F. Sokoya, *Building Your Otolaryngology Practice*,
https://doi.org/10.1007/978-3-032-27397-0_5

True productivity optimization is not about squeezing more work into the day. It is about removing friction so effort translates into output instead of waste.

Clinic Templates: The Architecture of Your Day

Clinic templates look mundane. They are anything but.

A template encodes assumptions about patient complexity, support staff availability, documentation burden, and whether access or depth is prioritized. When those assumptions do not match reality, inefficiency becomes invisible and normalized.

Early-career physicians often inherit templates designed for someone else. They assume inefficiency is personal rather than structural. Over time, they adapt to friction instead of questioning it.

That adaptation is costly.

A volume-heavy template without support pushes documentation into nights. A depth-heavy template without access throttles growth. A rigid template that doesn't evolve as your practice matures quietly drains energy.

The right template is not "busy." It is balanced, matched to your case mix and resources—and revisited periodically as your role changes.

Access Is a Throughput Variable, Not a Courtesy

Access is often framed as a patient-experience issue. In reality, it is a core productivity lever.

When referring physicians cannot get patients in, they route around you. When patients wait weeks for evaluation, downstream surgical volume suffers. When urgent cases become administrative battles, momentum is lost.

Availability does not mean chaos. It means intentional capacity—protected new-patient slots, add-on pathways, and staff empowered to move quickly when needed.

Practices that grow sustainably treat access as infrastructure, not generosity.

Documentation, "Pajama Time," and the Hidden Tax on Productivity

One of the most corrosive drains on productivity does not appear on the clinic schedule or OR board. It shows up at night.

Electronic health records have allowed us to quantify something physicians have complained about for years: work done after hours. This is often referred to as *"pajama time"*—documentation, chart review, and inbox management completed outside scheduled clinical hours.

Time-motion studies and EHR log analyses show that physicians spend substantial time on EHR work beyond face-to-face care, including evenings and weekends, and that this clerical burden is strongly associated with burnout and lower professional satisfaction [1, 2]. Importantly, this burden is not evenly distributed. Some physicians finish their workday relatively cleanly. Others carry it home every night.

The difference is rarely typing speed or discipline.

It is documentation structure.

When documentation is treated as an individual responsibility, the burden inevitably shifts onto the physician. When it is treated as a team function, the burden can be redistributed—and reduced.

Studies demonstrate that team-based documentation support, when implemented meaningfully, reduces physician documentation time and increases clinical throughput. In one EHR-based analysis, physicians whose notes were largely authored by team members—scribes, nurses, or medical assistants—spent significantly less time documenting and were able to see more patients per session [3]. By contrast, minimal or symbolic support had little impact; the work simply flowed back to the physician.

Support that does not materially change where the work is done does not improve productivity. It only changes who absorbs the inefficiency.

Support staff can amplify productivity—or create new bottlenecks.

APPs function as leverage when they independently manage post-ops, global visits, procedures, and clinics. When they are used primarily as shadows or scribes, they add overhead without reducing physician burden.

The same principle applies to coordinators, MAs, and schedulers. Every role must have a clear purpose tied to outcomes.

Productivity improves when support is intentional.

AI Transcription: A Practical Shift, Not a Panacea

Not every practice can support live scribes. Staffing costs, space constraints, or institutional resistance often make traditional scribe models difficult.

This is where AI-based ambient transcription tools have become relevant.

Recent studies suggest that high-quality ambient AI documentation can meaningfully reduce documentation burden and after-hours EHR time, particularly when physicians shift into an editor role rather than creating notes from scratch [4]. These tools are not perfect. They require oversight. They do not eliminate responsibility.

But they change the center of gravity.

Instead of building notes from nothing, physicians review, refine, and sign. For many, that difference alone is enough to reclaim evenings and weekends.

The lesson is not that AI solves everything. It's that documentation must be engineered, not endured. Whether the solution is a scribe, a trained MA, or AI, the goal is the same: reduce the amount of clerical work that only a physician can do.

If your productivity depends on work done at 10 p.m., it is not productivity—it is deferred cost.

OR Time: The Hardest Bottleneck to Fix

For procedural specialists, operating room time is often the tightest constraint on productivity—and the most misunderstood.

From the surgeon's perspective, OR inefficiency feels personal: late starts, slow turnovers, unavailable staff, block time that evaporates, cases bumped or delayed. The instinctive response is frustration, often directed at anesthesia, nursing, or administration.

Serving as Chief of Surgery fundamentally changed how I see this problem.

From a leadership perspective, OR inefficiency is rarely a single failure. It is a multi-variable coordination problem with competing incentives at every layer. The operating room sits at the intersection of staffing constraints, anesthesia availability, supply chain logistics, case-mix variability, PACU flow, bed capacity, union rules, and hospital-wide financial pressures.

Optimizing one variable often destabilizes another.

Increasing block utilization for one service line may worsen access for another. Speeding turnovers can stress nursing ratios. Pushing first-case on-time starts can conflict with anesthesia coverage realities. From the system's standpoint, the OR is not just a clinical workspace—it is a financial engine that must keep running, even when conditions are imperfect.

Understanding this doesn't excuse inefficiency—but it changes how you approach it.

High-functioning surgeons learn to think about OR productivity less in terms of ideal conditions and more in terms of constraint navigation. They are intentional about where cases are done, how complexity aligns with facility capability, and which cases tolerate variability.

As Dr. Young noted from experience across multiple sites, *"Where you operate matters as much as what you operate on."*

Surgeons who ignore this reality feel perpetually blocked. Surgeons who learn it gain leverage.

Metrics as Feedback, Not Judgment

Every system tracks metrics. Not all deserve equal attention.

Early in practice, the most useful metrics are local and directional:

- New-patient volume trends
- Stability of referral sources

- Clinic access lead times
- OR utilization and cancellation rates
- Productivity relative to support, not effort

Metrics are not moral judgments. They are feedback. Used properly, they identify bottlenecks before frustration sets in.

Burnout and Sustainability

Burnout is often framed as an emotional or resilience problem. Operationally, it is frequently a design failure.

When templates mismatch case mix, when access is constrained, when documentation spills into nights, and when OR time is unreliable, even highly motivated physicians erode.

Optimizing productivity is not about pushing harder. It is about aligning systems with reality so effort produces output rather than exhaustion. Productivity optimization is not about maximizing output this year. It is about creating a pace you can sustain for decades.

The practices that endure are not the ones that burn hottest. They are the ones that respect time as the limiting resource and design around it.

Bibliography

1. Sinsky C, et al. Allocation of physician time in ambulatory practice: a time and motion study in four specialties. Ann Intern Med. 2016;165(11):753–60.
2. Shanafelt TD, et al. Relationship between clerical burden and characteristics of the electronic environment with physician burnout and professional satisfaction. Mayo Clin Proc. 2016;91(7):836–48.
3. Apathy NC, Holmgren AJ, Cross DA. Physician EHR time and visit volume following adoption of team-based documentation support. JAMA Intern Med. 2024;184(10):1212–21.
4. Moy AJ, et al. Effect of ambient clinical documentation on physician documentation time and experience. JAMA. 2023.

6 Research and Innovation

Research is often framed as a fork in the road.

On one path is the clinician—busy, productive, practical. On the other is the academic—curious, investigative, theoretical. We're told, implicitly and sometimes explicitly, that we must choose. That once clinical volume ramps up, curiosity becomes a luxury.

That story doesn't hold up.

The evidence—and the lived experience of physicians with long, influential careers—points in a different direction: research, when done correctly, is not a distraction from practice building. It is one of the few things that makes long careers durable.

This chapter is about reclaiming research and innovation as tools—tools that buy meaning, leverage, and relevance in a system that increasingly reduces physicians to throughput.

Research as Meaning Infrastructure

Burnout is often discussed as a problem of workload. Increasingly, the literature frames it as a problem of *meaning*.

Large studies show that physicians who spend a meaningful portion of their professional time—roughly 20% or more—on the work they find most meaningful report lower burnout and higher professional fulfillment, even when overall work hours remain

F. Sokoya, *Building Your Otolaryngology Practice*,
https://doi.org/10.1007/978-3-032-27397-0_6

high [1]. In many cases, that meaningful work is research or teaching.

Research changes the texture of clinical work. It converts repetition into inquiry. It turns friction into questions. It gives clinicians a way to engage intellectually with problems that would otherwise feel draining.

This is why research-engaged physicians often describe their work as *sustaining* rather than exhausting—even when they are busy.

As Andrew Winkler reflected when describing his own trajectory in academic facial plastics:

> There are only so many years to work, and they go faster than you think. I always wanted to leave a mark.

Research, in this sense, isn't about padding a CV. It's about making the work feel worth doing 10, 15, 20 years in.

Research as Leverage Inside Systems

Modern healthcare systems run on metrics: RVUs, access, margins, throughput. In that environment, purely clinical value is increasingly commoditized.

Research changes that equation.

Faculty analyses from the AAMC and health-services literature consistently show that physicians with sustained scholarly output are more likely to hold leadership roles, retain protected time, and influence institutional priorities [2]. During periods of restructuring or consolidation, these physicians are also more likely to be retained—not because institutions are sentimental, but because research creates non-fungible value.

Put simply: a clinician who produces RVUs is replaceable. A clinician who produces RVUs *and* intellectual capital is harder to marginalize.

There's also a psychological dimension. When your value to the system extends beyond throughput, negotiations change. You have leverage—not just financial, but structural.

Research buys you a second lane of relevance.

You Don't Need a Lab to Be Influential

One of the most paralyzing myths in medicine is that "real" research requires a laboratory, grant funding, and protected time.

That may be true for bench science. It is not true for impact.

The modern literature makes this explicit. Clinical outcomes research, quality improvement, health-services research, and practice-based innovation now account for a large share of meaningful change in medicine [3]. Much of this work is driven by clinicians studying problems they encounter every day.

The National Academies' Learning Health System framework captures this well: care is delivered, outcomes are captured, the system learns, and practice improves—continuously [3]. Research is embedded in practice, not detached from it.

This is why the most productive research programs often begin with a simple question: *Why does this keep happening in my clinic?*

Henry Barham framed it in a way that strips away intimidation:

> You don't need permission to study what you're already doing.

Read generously, that statement isn't adversarial—it's liberating. It reframes research as something that grows *out of practice*, not something that competes with it.

And when the work is quality improvement—reducing complications, standardizing pathways, improving access—the SQUIRE 2.0 guidelines exist for a reason: they turn improvement work into scholarship the literature can trust [4].

What Makes Research "Productive"

Productive research is not defined by the number of publications. It is defined by what it reliably produces.

In practice, productive research generates one—or more—of the following:

- Better decisions: sharper indications, fewer gray zones
- Better outcomes: improvements patients can feel and you can measure
- Better systems: workflows that are repeatable, teachable, and scalable

Publications are one way to record these outputs. They are not the highest form of impact.

The highest leverage work is often what persists after the paper is forgotten: a protocol adopted across sites, a technique taught to trainees, a registry that quietly improves outcomes year after year.

That is research as infrastructure.

Innovation as Differentiation

In an era of increasing commoditization, differentiation matters.

Innovation—whether in technique, workflow, outcomes measurement, or patient experience—creates identity. It shifts referrals from convenience-based to intention-based. It changes how colleagues talk about you when your name comes up.

The diffusion-of-innovations literature shows that clinicians who generate and share practice-relevant insights disproportionately shape adoption patterns and professional norms [5]. Innovations spread not because they are true, but because they are adoptable—compatible with real workflows, supported by peers, and reinforced through professional networks [5].

Research, in this sense, is not just discovery. It is signal.

For those practicing in academic otolaryngology, it is also important to understand that "research" is not a single path, but a spectrum of formal tracks, each with different expectations and trade-offs. At the trainee level, T32 training grants support residents or fellows during protected research time, often serving as an entry point into academic investigation and signaling institutional commitment to scholarship. Early-career faculty may pursue career development *awards* (such as K-series grants), which provide mentored time to build independent research skills while maintaining a clinical footprint. More established investigators often compete for R-series grants, particularly the R01, which fund investigator-initiated research programs and confer substantial academic credibility and autonomy. Alongside these NIH mechanisms, many otolaryngologists engage in foundation grants, industry-sponsored studies, outcomes research, or health-services research that may not require large federal funding but still meaningfully advance the field. The key point is that each pathway carries different implications for protected time, clinical expectations, and career identity. Understanding these distinctions early allows physicians to choose a research trajectory that aligns with their interests and tolerance for risk, rather than drifting into a model whose demands they did not anticipate.

Teaching Multiplies Impact

For many physicians, the most enduring legacy is not a paper. It's a person.

Teaching multiplies research by transferring judgment. It's not about slides or lectures; it's about *taste*—how you think, how you decide, what you tolerate, what you never compromise on.

Winkler described this ripple effect when reflecting on his mentor:

> Ted Cook trained dozens of fellows. Many of them went on to start their own programs. His impact spread far beyond anything he did himself.

That's the compounding effect. A paper is a snapshot. A trainee is a multiplier.

The most durable research programs use teaching as their distribution channel. You don't just publish a technique—you teach it, standardize it, and embed it into culture. That's how innovations stick.

The Long View

Research is not a detour from practice building. It is part of it.

It buys meaning when volume alone would hollow you out. It buys leverage when systems tighten. It buys durability when careers stretch long. You do not need an academic title to benefit from it. You need curiosity, discipline, and the willingness to ask better questions about the work you're already doing.

Curiosity, structured and sustained, becomes endurance.

What often goes unsaid is how deeply these research pathways shape promotion and tenure—not just in theory, but in lived experience. In most academic otolaryngology departments, advancement is less about any single paper or grant and more about demonstrating a coherent scholarly identity over time. Promotion committees look for trajectory: evidence that your work is building toward something larger, that your contributions are recognizable, and that your impact extends beyond your clinic walls. For some, that coherence comes through NIH-funded discovery; for others, through sustained outcomes research, educational scholarship, guideline development, or national leadership tied to innovation. The aspirational goal is not to check boxes, but to become known for something that matters. When research, teaching, and clinical work reinforce one another, promotion becomes a natural consequence rather than a forced campaign—and tenure, where it exists, becomes less about security and more about the freedom to pursue ideas that shape the field for the next generation.

Bibliography

1. Shanafelt TD, et al. Impact of organizational leadership on physician burnout and satisfaction. Mayo Clin Proc. 2015;90(4):432–40.
2. AAMC. The role of scholarship in faculty advancement and retention. AAMC Analysis; 2022.
3. National Academies of Sciences, Engineering, and Medicine. Best care at lower cost: the path to continuously learning health care in America. 2013.
4. Ogrinc G, et al. SQUIRE 2.0 (standards for quality improvement reporting excellence). BMJ Qual Saf. 2016;25(12):986–92.
5. Greenhalgh T, et al. Diffusion of innovations in health service organizations. Milbank Q. 2004;82(4):581–629.

7 Negotiating Contracts

Chris Voss is a former FBI hostage negotiator, and the author of *Never Split the Difference*, a book grounded in real-world negotiations where mistakes carried immediate and irreversible consequences. Unlike traditional business negotiation frameworks that emphasize compromise or persuasion, Voss's approach is built around psychological realism—how people actually behave under pressure, with asymmetric power and incomplete information. That perspective maps uncomfortably well onto physician contract negotiations, where timelines are compressed, information is uneven, and risk is often transferred quietly rather than explicitly discussed. Voss's framework is valuable here not because it promises dominance, but because it teaches physicians how to recognize leverage, uncover hidden costs, and avoid agreements that appear reasonable but create long-term exposure.

Most physicians believe negotiation begins when the offer letter arrives.

That's already too late.

By the time a contract hits your inbox, the institution has already decided how you will be used, how replaceable you are, and where risk will sit if things don't work out. The document in front of you is not an invitation to negotiate from scratch—it is a reflection of assumptions already made.

Contracts are not legal documents first. They are behavioral documents. They encode incentives. They determine who absorbs

F. Sokoya, *Building Your Otolaryngology Practice*, https://doi.org/10.1007/978-3-032-27397-0_7

friction, who carries risk, and how your days will unfold long after the excitement of a new job fades.

This chapter is about learning to read contracts the way institutions do—and negotiating with clarity instead of hope.

Why Physicians Negotiate the Wrong Things

Early-career physicians tend to fixate on what feels tangible: base salary, signing bonus, relocation allowance. These are easy to compare and emotionally satisfying to improve.

Institutions know this.

They are often willing to adjust headline numbers if it secures agreement on the terms that matter more over time: productivity expectations, staffing ratios, termination clauses, non-competes, and control over schedule and scope.

Many physicians "win" the salary negotiation and quietly lose the job.

The loss rarely shows up in year one. It reveals itself in year three, when expectations rise, support lags, and flexibility disappears.

Leverage Is Not Assertiveness. It's Asymmetry

Physicians often misunderstand leverage.

They think leverage comes from confidence, clever arguments, or having a strong lawyer. In reality, leverage comes from asymmetry—when the cost of losing you is higher than the cost of losing them.

Voss is explicit about this: leverage exists when one party has real alternatives and the other does not.

In medicine, leverage is rarely created at the table. It is created beforehand through:

- Reputation that drives referrals.
- Skills that are scarce locally.
- Productivity that solves institutional problems.

- Breadth that prevents easy substitution.
- Optionality—the credible ability to walk away.

This is why negotiation feels frustrating early in a career. You are trying to *argue* your way into leverage instead of *building* your way into it.

As Voss puts it, leverage comes from being able to say no—and meaning it.

So What Leverage Do you Actually Have as a New Graduate?

This is the uncomfortable question every resident and fellow is thinking: *What leverage do I really have right now?*

The honest answer is this: you don't yet have positional leverage—but you do have structural leverage.

You may not have an established referral base or years of productivity data, but you do have things institutions value:

- Current, in-demand skills that are difficult to recruit.
- Time and flexibility senior physicians no longer have.
- Lower political friction within the system.
- The ability to grow into problems the institution already has.

Hospitals and groups are not hiring you for what you've already built. They are hiring you for what they believe you can become.

That belief is leverage.

As a new residency or fellowship graduate, your leverage often lies in geographic placement and site assignment, initial scope of practice, early support structures (APPs, scribes, clinic templates), and protected time to build clinics, programs, or skills.

You replace reputation with clarity. Institutions respond to candidates who understand their problems and articulate how they can help solve them.

Your leverage is not who you are today.

It is who you can become *inside their system*—and whether they believe you.

Contracts Are Systems, Not Lists

One of the most common mistakes physicians make is treating contracts as a checklist: salary, RVU rate, call, non-compete.

That's not how institutions think.

Contracts are systems. Changing one variable changes the value of the others.

Voss emphasizes this repeatedly: negotiation is not about winning points—it's about reshaping the deal landscape.

A lower base salary may be acceptable if RVU conversion is favorable and thresholds are realistic.

A broader non-compete may be tolerable if termination requires longer notice and tail coverage is paid.

A heavier call burden may be reasonable if call is compensated and post-call expectations are explicit.

Nothing is sacred. Everything is tradeable.

The mistake is negotiating each clause in isolation. The skill is understanding what you are giving up—and what you are buying in return.

As Voss notes, the deal is not the price. The deal is the terms.

Compensation Structures: Who Carries the Risk?

Every compensation model answers the same question: *who carries the risk?*

High base salaries with low productivity conversion often shift risk to you later. Pure RVU models reward volume but can punish complexity. Collections models expose you to payer mix and overhead. Hybrids often look fair until thresholds quietly rise.

You are not negotiating pay alone. You are negotiating friction.

Ask yourself:

- What happens if I exceed expectations?
- What happens if I don't?
- Who controls the variables that determine my income?

If the answer is "not me," proceed carefully.

Insurance, Tail Coverage, and Hidden Career Risk

Salary gets attention. Insurance determines freedom.

Most physician contracts provide claims-made malpractice insurance, not occurrence-based coverage. Under claims-made policies, coverage applies only if the policy is active when the claim is filed—not when the care occurred.

That means when you leave a job, someone must purchase tail coverage to protect you against future claims arising from past work.

Tail coverage is expensive. It commonly costs 1.5–2 times your annual malpractice premium, often payable as a lump sum. Many contracts quietly assign that responsibility to the physician.

This is not accidental. It is risk transfer.

Tail coverage interacts with other clauses in ways that materially affect your freedom:

- A short termination notice plus physician-paid tail creates financial shock.
- A broad non-compete plus physician-paid tail can function as a trap.
- For-cause termination language that triggers tail responsibility increases asymmetry.

Physicians often discover this only when they try to leave—when the cost of exit becomes painfully real.

Voss's concept of loss aversion applies perfectly here. Humans tolerate bad conditions to avoid large, immediate losses. Tail coverage exploits that instinct.

Negotiation here is not about confrontation. It is about foresight:

- What type of malpractice policy is provided?
- Who pays for tail, and under what circumstances?
- How does tail interact with termination and non-compete language?

If the answers are vague, the risk is yours.

Calibrated Questions: How to Uncover the Truth

Voss teaches that the goal of negotiation is not agreement—it is truth.

Calibrated questions—*how* and *what* questions—force the other side to solve the problem for you. They reveal assumptions without accusation.

Questions physicians should ask include:

- *How does the system support physicians who exceed expectations?*
- *What happens if clinic demand outpaces staffing?*
- *How have others exited this role, and what did that look like?*
- *How do you see this role evolving over five years?*

As Voss says, your goal is not to get to yes. Your goal is to understand what you are agreeing to.

Walking Away Is a Skill

Not every contract should be signed.

This is difficult advice for physicians conditioned to be selected rather than select. But walking away from a bad deal is often the strongest move you can make.

Walking away does not mean burning bridges. It means being clear, professional, and aligned with your long-term trajectory.

Remember the opening line: no deal is better than a bad deal.

Process of Gathering Information

The more information you have the better. Ask yourself this questions:

What are the challenges?
What gaps are they trying to fill?
What's the current landscape?
Do they have a pool of money set aside for student loan repayment but they're not volunteering that information?

Reducing information asymmetry is key to strong negotiations.

Contracts feel intimidating because they arrive at a moment of transition.

You have spent years proving that you belong in the room—through exams, call nights, long cases, and constant evaluation. When the first real offer arrives, the natural instinct is relief. A job. Stability. A place to begin.

But contracts are not celebrations. They are architecture.

They determine how risk is distributed, how effort is rewarded, how autonomy expands or contracts, and how easy it will be to leave if the arrangement stops working. Most physicians only discover this after the excitement fades—when the daily realities of a job begin to surface.

Negotiation, in this sense, is not about winning. It is about clarity.

You are not trying to defeat the other side. You are trying to understand what you are agreeing to—and whether that agreement aligns with the life you intend to build. Sometimes the answer will be yes. Sometimes the answer will be no. Both outcomes are valuable.

Chris Voss often reminds negotiators that the most powerful word in a negotiation is no. Not because saying no ends conversations, but because it forces honesty. It reveals where the boundaries are, what is actually flexible, and whether the deal makes sense at all.

Physicians are conditioned to avoid that moment. We are trained to accommodate, to adapt, to make things work. Those instincts serve patients well. They serve contracts less well.

The goal is not to become adversarial. The goal is to become deliberate.

A well-negotiated contract does not guarantee a perfect job. Systems change, leadership turns over, and incentives evolve. But a clear contract protects you from surprises and preserves the ability to adapt when circumstances shift.

That protection is not about money alone. It is about agency.

Because in the end, the purpose of negotiating a contract is not to maximize the first year of your career. It is to ensure that the path you are stepping onto remains one you are free to shape.

And that freedom is worth negotiating for.

8 Academic Practice

Academic medicine occupies a strange place in the collective imagination of physicians.

It is often described in moral terms—noble, mission-driven, intellectually pure—or dismissed as inefficient, political, and underpaid. Both caricatures are partially true.

Academic practice is neither inherently virtuous nor inherently flawed. It is a system, and like all systems, it rewards certain behaviors while punishing others.

This chapter is not about whether academic medicine is "good" or "bad." It is about understanding why some physicians thrive in it, while others leave disillusioned—and how to tell which outcome is more likely for you.

To do that, we will examine three case studies. They were chosen deliberately.

Andrew Winkler and *Yadro Ducic* were formative mentors during residency and fellowship—surgeons who demonstrated what high-level academic practice *can* look like when autonomy, rigor, and standards are preserved. *Oswaldo Henriquez* represents a different but equally important arc: a surgeon who built a successful academic practice and then deliberately transitioned into a community-based model—carrying academic standards with him.

Together, they illustrate not a single "right" way to practice academically, but a set of principles that determine whether academic medicine becomes a platform or a trap.

F. Sokoya, *Building Your Otolaryngology Practice*,
https://doi.org/10.1007/978-3-032-27397-0_8

What Academic Medicine Actually Optimizes For

Before examining individual paths, it's important to understand what academic systems are designed to optimize.

Despite the language of mission, most academic medical centers are structurally optimized around:

- Clinical throughput.
- Institutional reputation.
- Teaching capacity.
- Grant and publication output.
- Service-line stability.

What they do *not* reliably optimize for is individual physician autonomy.

This mismatch is the source of much academic dissatisfaction. Physicians enter expecting freedom of thought and intellectual exploration, and instead encounter productivity targets, access pressures, and administrative constraints that feel indistinguishable from employed practice—often without the same financial upside.

The difference between thriving and burning out in academia lies in whether you can align your personal goals with what the system actually rewards.

Case Study I: Yadro Ducic—Academic Rigor Without Academic Dependency

Yadro Ducic's career is instructive precisely because it breaks the mental model most physicians inherit about academic success.

In 1997, he established his practice in the Dallas–Fort Worth metroplex—at a time when high-level head and neck oncology with microvascular free tissue transfer was still largely concentrated within university hospitals. He did not rely on an academic appointment for credibility, referrals, or platform.

Instead, he built one.

From the outset, Ducic practiced at a level that would have been indistinguishable from any major academic center: complex head and neck oncologic surgery, advanced microvascular reconstruction, and a full spectrum of facial plastic and reconstructive procedures. He treated tertiary- and quaternary-level disease in a community setting, drawing referrals not because of institutional branding, but because outcomes spoke for themselves.

What followed over the next two decades is difficult to overstate.

Ducic published more than 200 peer-reviewed manuscripts, many of them shaping modern reconstructive paradigms in head and neck surgery. He trained over 20 head and neck oncologic, microvascular and facial plastic fellows, many of whom went on to lead programs, build practices, and train others in turn. His influence propagated outward—not through a department chair title, but through standards, technique, and expectation.

And he did all of this without working for a university.

That distinction matters. Ducic's career demonstrates that academic credibility is not conferred by payroll status. It is earned through rigor, consistency, and contribution. His work met academic standards because he imposed those standards on himself and his trainees, not because an institution required it.

This model carries an uncomfortable implication for physicians considering academic medicine: the institution is not the source of intellectual authority. It can be a vehicle—but it is not a prerequisite.

Ducic's path also highlights something more subtle. Because his value was rooted in expertise rather than affiliation, his autonomy was unusually durable. He controlled scope, pace, and evolution of his practice. His academic output did not compete with his clinical work; it grew out of it.

For physicians wrestling with whether academic medicine is the "only" path to scholarly impact, Ducic's career offers a counterexample that is both liberating and demanding. It shows what is possible when academic standards are treated as a personal commitment rather than an institutional obligation.

Case Study II: Andrew Winkler—Building Something Real inside Academia

If Ducic's career demonstrates academic rigor without institutional dependence, Andrew Winkler's career demonstrates something just as rare: how to build an authentic, high-functioning academic practice from the inside—without surrendering autonomy.

When Winkler joined the University of Colorado, he was not stepping into a fully formed division with established resources and a clear mandate. He was, in many ways, starting a program from scratch. Facial plastic surgery existed nominally within the department, but it was not yet a coherent, self-sustaining entity with a defined identity, scope, or growth strategy.

What followed over the next decade was not accidental.

Winkler worked—hard. He built clinical volume deliberately, taking on complex reconstructive cases while simultaneously pushing the boundaries of what could be done within an academic environment on the aesthetic side. Rather than accepting the implicit academic narrative that cosmetic surgery was peripheral or incompatible with scholarship, he demonstrated—through outcomes and demand—that high-level cosmetic facial plastic surgery could coexist with resident education, research, and institutional mission.

That coexistence required intentionality. Winkler understood early that if facial plastics was going to thrive academically, it could not simply be absorbed into the general ENT workflow. It needed its own standards, its own expectations, and eventually its own identity. He focused on creating a clinical environment that matched patient expectations for aesthetic care while remaining integrated within the academic system—a balance many fail to strike.

At the same time, he committed deeply to education. For over a decade, Winkler trained residents in facial plastic and reconstructive surgery, transmitting not just technique, but judgment. Residents learned how to think through cases, how to balance form and function, and how to operate at a level that did not require constant supervision. Teaching was not an add-on; it was part of the division's DNA.

As the practice grew, Winkler faced one of the most difficult challenges in academic medicine: partner selection. Growth brings risk. Hiring the wrong person can fracture a division; hiring the right one can multiply it.

Winkler was deliberate. He prioritized work ethic, technical excellence, and cultural fit. He understood that autonomy only survives when partners are aligned in values. As new attendings joined, he encouraged them to explore and develop their own interests rather than forcing them into predefined roles. That freedom was not indulgent—it was strategic. Physicians who feel ownership over their work are more productive, more loyal, and more invested.

Over time, the division grew into a four-attending facial plastic surgery group, each with distinct strengths but shared standards. With that critical mass in place, Winkler took the next step: building a fellowship program. The fellowship was not created to inflate prestige. It was created to formalize teaching, extend the division's reach, and ensure continuity of standards beyond any single individual.

Perhaps most importantly, Winkler preserved autonomy at each stage. He stayed in academia not out of inertia, but because the environment continued to allow him to shape his own career. When leadership supported physician-driven growth and compensation structures rewarded effort, academic medicine became a platform rather than a constraint.

Winkler's career illustrates a crucial lesson for physicians considering academia: it is possible to push the limits of what an academic environment allows—but only if you are willing to build, not wait. Autonomy is rarely granted in academia. It is earned through value creation, credibility, and sustained contribution.

For those who believe academic medicine must inevitably dilute ambition, Winkler's example offers a counterpoint. Academia can work—but only when physicians are willing to define it on their own terms.

Case Study III: Oswaldo Henriquez—Carrying Academic Rigor into the Community

If Ducic represents academic rigor without institutional dependency, and Winkler represents academic rigor successfully cultivated from within, Oswaldo Henriquez represents a third, equally important path: academic excellence that evolves deliberately into the community setting.

Henriquez spent years practicing at Grady Memorial Hospital, one of the most demanding safety-net hospitals in the country. In that environment, there was no room for superficial competence. The pathology was real, the resources were constrained, and the margin for error was small. He treated complex patients with advanced disease, many of whom had nowhere else to go.

During that time, Henriquez served as a core educator in a setting where theory met consequence. Residents learned not just how to operate, but how to think under pressure—how to triage, how to adapt when ideal conditions didn't exist, and how to maintain standards even when the system made that difficult. Teaching was not protected time; it was woven into the work itself.

Clinically, Henriquez built a practice defined by breadth and rigor. He became a regional authority in facial trauma, helping to pioneer and refine approaches to complex craniofacial injuries in a high-volume, real-world setting. At the same time, he continued to advance skills in rhinology and skull base surgery, maintaining a scope of practice that resisted early narrowing. This breadth was not accidental. It was strategic—insulating his practice from overspecialization while expanding his value to the system.

He published consistently, contributed to the literature, and participated in multidisciplinary care at a level indistinguishable from any traditional academic center. His credibility came from outcomes and consistency, not from title alone.

Over time, however, Henriquez recognized a familiar tension: the ceiling he was experiencing was structural, not personal. Autonomy over schedule, scope, and growth was increasingly constrained—not by lack of skill or ambition, but by the architecture of the institution itself.

The decision to move into a community-based practice was therefore not reactive. It was deliberate.

In the community setting, Henriquez did not abandon academic standards. He carried them with him. He applied the same rigor to case selection, operative planning, multidisciplinary collaboration, and outcomes awareness. What changed was not the quality of the work, but the degree of flexibility around how and when it was done.

That flexibility translated into renewed fulfillment. The ability to shape his practice more directly, to align effort with reward, and to grow without navigating layers of institutional inertia restored a sense of ownership that many academic physicians quietly miss.

Henriquez's path matters because it reframes a common false dichotomy. Leaving academia does not require lowering standards. It requires re-anchoring those standards to yourself rather than the institution.

His career demonstrates that academic medicine can be a destination, a foundation, or a phase—and that the skills developed there, when chosen intentionally, can thrive outside its walls. For physicians who fear that leaving academia means losing intellectual identity, Henriquez offers a counterexample: rigor is portable, if you choose to carry it.

Why Academic Physicians Leave

Most academic physicians do not leave because they dislike teaching or research.

They leave because of persistent misalignment—a growing gap between what the institution demands and what allows them to do their best work.

The most common inflection points are structural, not emotional.

Over time, many academic physicians experience a slow erosion of autonomy. Clinic templates become tighter without additional support. Productivity expectations rise while protected time quietly shrinks. Leadership changes introduce new priorities that reward visibility or volume over depth. What once felt like intellectual freedom begins to feel like constant negotiation for resources.

Another driver is role compression. Academic physicians are often asked to be excellent clinicians, committed teachers, productive researchers, and reliable administrators—without clear boundaries between those roles. When everything is a priority, nothing truly is. The result is chronic overextension without a sense of progress.

Compensation also plays a role, though rarely in isolation. Many physicians tolerate lower pay in exchange for mission and meaning. What becomes intolerable is misaligned compensation—being asked to generate high clinical volume while also producing scholarship, without adequate recognition of either. Over time, that imbalance breeds resentment rather than fulfillment.

Perhaps most importantly, academic physicians leave when they realize that the ceiling they are hitting is structural rather than personal. When growth stalls not because of skill or ambition, but because of institutional architecture, leaving becomes an act of clarity rather than frustration.

Leaving academia, in this sense, is rarely a rejection of values. It is often a decision to preserve them.

At one point in my career, I had to confront a quiet dissonance. The version of academic medicine I had believed in—one that I had internalized through training and mentorship—no longer matched the reality I found myself practicing within. It is possible that I had changed. It is equally possible that my earlier assumptions were incomplete. In the end, it didn't matter which was true. What mattered was recognizing the misalignment and deciding to act on it. Leaving that environment felt, at the time, somewhere between bold and foolish. Academic medicine carries gravity, and stepping away from it can feel like abandoning a path you were trained to respect. But the experiment worked. Building a high-volume practice in head and neck oncology and facial plastic surgery outside the ivory tower turned out to be more intellectually engaging, professionally satisfying, and personally fulfilling than

I had allowed myself to imagine. What I thought I might lose in leaving, I ultimately rediscovered in a different form—autonomy, rigor, and the quiet satisfaction of building something that was truly my own.

Why Academic Physicians Stay

For those who remain—and thrive—academic medicine offers something difficult to replicate elsewhere.

At its best, academia provides intellectual oxygen. It creates space for inquiry, teaching, and contribution beyond the individual patient encounter. Physicians who stay often do so because their curiosity is rewarded rather than tolerated.

Teaching is a powerful anchor. Many academic physicians derive deep meaning from shaping the next generation—transmitting judgment, standards, and professional identity in ways that extend far beyond their own careers. The ripple effect of mentorship can be more satisfying than any individual achievement.

Research and innovation also keep physicians engaged over decades. When scholarship aligns with clinical work—when questions arise naturally from practice and feed back into better care—academic medicine becomes energizing rather than draining. The work evolves instead of repeating.

Leadership is another reason physicians stay. Academic environments can offer pathways to influence policy, shape programs, and define standards at a regional or national level. For physicians motivated by impact beyond their own clinic, this platform matters.

Finally, academic physicians stay when the environment gets out of the way. Supportive leadership, transparent expectations, and respect for physician-driven growth transform academia from a constraint into a multiplier. In those settings, autonomy is not absolute—but it is sufficient.

Staying in academia is not about tolerance. It is about alignment.

The Underlying Truth

Academic medicine does not fail people. Misalignment does.

Physicians who leave are not weaker. Physicians who stay are not purer. Both groups are responding rationally to the incentives and constraints around them.

The lesson for the reader is not to choose academia or avoid it. The lesson is to understand what academic systems actually reward, and to decide—clearly and honestly—whether those rewards align with the life and career you want to build.

When that alignment exists, academic medicine can be a lifelong platform.

When it does not, leaving can be the most professional decision you make.

9 Hospital-Employed Practice

Jon Young chose hospital employment deliberately.

He wanted infrastructure—multidisciplinary teams, OR access for complex pediatric cases, and a referral network that would have taken years to build independently. A large multispecialty system offered all of that on day one. The decision was rational and, for many physicians, it would have been the obvious one.

What the offer letter did not describe was everything else.

Over time, Young encountered the hidden architecture of hospital-employed practice: access expectations that turned trust into triple-booked clinics, metrics that measured activity more easily than judgment, and institutional priorities that did not always align with how he wanted to build his career. None of this was malicious. It was structural. And it is the reality that most hospital-employed physicians eventually discover—often after the initial relief of a stable job has faded.

Young's response to that reality is what makes his career instructive. He did not leave. He did not comply passively. He learned how the system worked, positioned himself where his contribution was visible and hard to replicate, and built programs from the inside that outlasted any single leadership cycle.

His story is not about hospital employment being good or bad. It is about what it actually takes to practice well inside one.

F. Sokoya, *Building Your Otolaryngology Practice*,
https://doi.org/10.1007/978-3-032-27397-0_9

What Hospital Employment Actually Is

Even when physicians believe they are joining "a group," the group is often part of a system. Even when the logo says "medical group," the incentives are hospital incentives. Hospital systems are large, complex enterprises under margin pressure and public scrutiny. They run on measurable signals: access, throughput, quality dashboards, standardized workflows, and patient experience scores.

To thrive in hospital-employed practice, you have to understand one thing early: you are operating inside a corporate structure. That is not cynicism. It is description. And once you see it clearly, you can stop being surprised by the rules.

The language changes first. "Patients" become "consumers." "Physicians" become "providers." "Clinic time" becomes "capacity." Then the expectations follow.

Most young physicians assume hospital employment means "less business, more medicine." Sometimes it does. More often, it changes where business pressure expresses itself. Instead of worrying about payroll and rent, you experience it through clinic access expectations, template pressure, OR utilization targets, documentation requirements, prior authorization workflows, and staffing volatility.

Hospital employment does not remove economics from your life. It changes its form.

This is why the same contract can feel supportive in one environment and suffocating in another. The paper is not the whole job. The environment is.

Goodhart's Law in Medicine

Goodhart's Law is simple: when a measure becomes a target, it stops being a good measure. That is not cynicism—it is how systems behave under pressure.

Hospital systems need ways to track performance across hundreds of physicians and dozens of service lines. So they measure.

They measure access and capacity—how quickly new patients can be seen, how many open slots exist, whether you are the bottleneck. They measure throughput—visits per session, procedure conversion, OR utilization, turnover time. They measure quality—readmissions, safety events, infections, standardization. And they measure patient experience.

None of this is inherently wrong. Measurement creates accountability. It identifies gaps. It drives improvement.

The problem begins when measurement becomes the mission.

Patient experience scores illustrate this most clearly. Hospitals adopted tools like Net Promoter Score and HCAHPS surveys for legitimate reasons: to give patients a voice, to make performance transparent, and to create incentives for improvement. NPS measures loyalty and likelihood to recommend. HCAHPS, mandated by CMS, standardizes patient experience reporting and ties it to public reporting and value-based purchasing [1–3].

When these scores function as signals—diagnostic tools that highlight communication gaps, chaotic discharge processes, or understaffed units—they improve care. The problem is that once scores are tied to dashboards, incentives, and departmental accountability, the organization naturally starts optimizing for the number rather than the thing the number was meant to represent.

Three patterns tend to follow.

First, patient experience becomes confused with clinical quality. Many drivers of satisfaction scores are not clinical—parking, wait time, billing confusion, front-desk interactions. Good care can score poorly if the experience is inconvenient. Poor care can score well if the experience is polished.

Second, difficult medicine gets penalized. The sickest patients are not always "promoters," even when cared for expertly. Honest conversations about uncertainty, risks, or prognosis rarely feel good in the moment. When scores become targets, the system implicitly nudges clinicians toward what preserves satisfaction today rather than what protects outcomes tomorrow.

Third, behavior drifts toward score protection. Subtle patterns emerge: reluctance to take complex or unhappy patients, pressure to smooth conversations, an overinvestment in optics, and a quiet erosion of physician judgment in favor of customer-service scripting.

This is Goodhart's Law enacted at institutional scale.

The solution is not to dismiss patient experience. It is to keep it in its proper place—as one signal among many, interpreted with context. Patient experience matters, but it must never outrank clinical integrity. Hospitals that get this right use experience data to diagnose operational friction, not to coerce physicians into practicing with a retail mindset.

Young described the tension plainly. Access, he noted, becomes "the tax of being trusted"—and in some systems that trust results in triple-booked clinics to protect referral relationships. The metric says you are succeeding. The lived experience says you are drowning. Learning to distinguish between the two is essential.

How Young Built Inside the System

Young did not enter hospital employment passively. From early on, he treated the system as a platform rather than a destination.

When he identified unmet needs—pediatric airway cases that no one wanted, craniofacial work that required coordination across multiple services—he filled them. Not because the system asked, but because the gaps were obvious and he was willing to own the complexity.

That willingness created leverage.

Over time, Young became the physician other departments relied on for cases that did not fit neatly into anyone else's scope. That breadth—pediatric airway, craniofacial, multidisciplinary care—was not accidental. It was strategic. It made him difficult to replace and gave him standing to advocate for resources, staffing, and program development in ways that a narrower clinical profile would not have supported.

He also learned something that many hospital-employed physicians discover too late: influence inside a system does not come from formal authority. It comes from solving problems that the system recognizes but cannot easily fix on its own. Young's growth within his organization came not from titles or committees, but from being the person others trusted to handle complexity when no one else would.

That trust translated into practical autonomy—not absolute, but sufficient. He shaped his clinical scope, influenced how cases were distributed, and built programs that outlasted any single leadership cycle.

His example counters a common narrative: that hospital employment inevitably reduces physicians to interchangeable production units. It can. But it does not have to—if you understand what the system values and position yourself where your contribution is visible and hard to replicate.

The Corporate Trade-Off: Convenience in Exchange for Control

Hospital employment offers something undeniably attractive: relief from the mechanics of running a business. Payroll is handled. Contracts are negotiated at scale. Capital expenditures are no longer personal decisions. Marketing, compliance, IT, and billing fade into the background.

For many physicians, especially early in their careers, this feels like freedom.

But it is not free.

What hospital employment really does is exchange one set of burdens for another. You are relieved of financial and operational risk, but in return you cede control over the levers that shape your daily work. The practice no longer belongs to you in any meaningful sense; it belongs to the system, and you operate within its priorities.

That lack of control often shows up subtly at first. Clinic templates tighten. Scheduling rules standardize. Staffing becomes variable rather than bespoke. Decisions that once required a conversation now require a committee. Over time, the distance between effort and outcome grows. You work harder, but the sense of ownership shrinks.

At the same time, hospital employment provides real advantages that should not be minimized. Scale matters. Payer contracts are stronger. Facilities are accessible. Referral pipelines are broader. Programs that would take years to build independently can be launched quickly with institutional backing. For complex, multidisciplinary care—the kind Young built his career around—this infrastructure is not just helpful. It is often essential.

This is the trade-off.

You gain insulation from risk, but you lose discretion. You gain convenience, but you surrender authorship. Your success becomes increasingly dependent on how well you function inside a system rather than how well you design your own.

Physicians who thrive in hospital-employed practice are not the ones who deny this trade-off. They are the ones who understand it early and negotiate around it—preserving control where it matters most, staying involved in governance, and refusing to outsource judgment entirely.

Those who struggle are often those who believed employment meant freedom from business, only to discover that corporate priorities did not eliminate business pressure—they simply relocated it.

Hospital employment can be a platform. It can also become a cage. The difference lies in whether you recognize what you have traded away—and whether you are intentional about what you keep.

How to Thrive in Hospital-Employed Practice Without Losing Yourself

The paradox of modern hospital-employed practice is this: the more corporate medicine becomes, the more valuable old-school medicine actually is.

Not because it resists metrics—but because it anchors judgment.

Old-school medicine is not about ignoring data or rejecting systems. It is about remembering that trust, reliability, and clinical integrity are not fully capturable by dashboards. These qualities still drive referrals, loyalty, and reputation, even when they do not show up neatly on a spreadsheet.

Physicians who thrive inside hospital systems learn to perform well in the measured world without allowing measurement to replace meaning.

They understand the metrics. They respect them. They do not dismiss them. But they also know which parts of medicine cannot be outsourced to surveys or scores: showing up when it matters, taking ownership of outcomes, communicating clearly when the answer is difficult, and earning trust over time rather than optimizing for the moment.

This is where old-school values quietly outperform corporate logic.

Reliability still matters. When you consistently return calls, take care of referrals, and follow through, people remember. Departments remember. Systems remember. These behaviors reduce friction in ways no policy ever will.

Judgment still matters. Knowing when to push forward and when to stop, when to reassure and when to be honest, when to operate and when not to—these decisions shape outcomes far more than any metric. High-functioning systems eventually recognize this, even if they struggle to measure it.

Relationships still matter. Hospital-employed physicians who invest in relationships—with colleagues, staff, administrators, and referring physicians—create informal networks of trust that protect them when metrics fluctuate or leadership changes. These relationships are often the difference between being supported and being scrutinized.

Most importantly, ownership still matters. Even when you do not own your practice, you can own your work. Physicians who treat their role as a craft rather than a job find ways to shape their environment—through committees, program building, mentorship, and leadership—rather than being shaped by it.

Thriving in hospital-employed practice is not about resisting the system. It is about operating with clarity inside it.

You learn the language of metrics without speaking it exclusively. You meet expectations without letting them define you. You build a reputation that outlasts dashboards and leadership cycles.

Old-school medicine was never about rejecting progress. It was about grounding progress in responsibility. That grounding is not obsolete. If anything, it is more valuable now than ever.

When you bring that mindset into corporate medicine, you stop feeling managed—and start feeling effective.

As Dr. Henriquez put it: "That is how hospital employment becomes a platform rather than a cage."

Bibliography

1. Centers for Medicare & Medicaid Services (CMS). Hospital CAHPS (HCAHPS). Updated Apr 21, 2025.
2. CMS. CAHPS surveys and value-based purchasing (Pay for Performance). Updated May 19, 2025; and Hospital Value-Based Purchasing Program. Updated Jun 3, 2025.
3. Press Ganey. Unlocking the power of NPS in healthcare (and related best practices). 2024–2025.

Private Practice 10

There is no such thing as *private practice*.

That phrase suggests a single model—a coherent alternative to academia or hospital employment. It implies that once you leave an institution, you enter a stable, defined category where autonomy, ownership, and independence naturally follow.

That belief is the source of most private practice disappointment.

Private practice is not a model. It is a container. What happens inside that container depends entirely on how it is designed, governed, financed, and led. Two practices can both call themselves "private" and function as completely different organisms—one durable and generative, the other brittle and exhausting.

This chapter is about learning to see private practice clearly, stripped of mythology.

There Is No One Version of "Private" Practice

Some practices function like boutiques—low volume, high margin, carefully controlled pace. Others resemble tightly run operational machines where efficiency and throughput are the dominant virtues. Some act as tertiary referral centers, built on complexity, reputation, and trust rather than speed. Others exist in hybrid

F. Sokoya, *Building Your Otolaryngology Practice*,
https://doi.org/10.1007/978-3-032-27397-0_10

alignment with hospitals, preserving clinical autonomy while offloading administrative burden.

Each of these behaves differently under stress. Each rewards different personalities. Each fails in different ways.

The mistake is assuming that choosing "private practice" is the decision. The real decision is which version of private practice you are building, and whether it matches who you are.

Physicians who thrive in private practice are not the ones chasing freedom. They are the ones designing constraint.

Private Practice Is a Margin Engine, Not a Volume Engine

One of the most persistent illusions about private practice is that success is a function of staying busy. Many practices fail not because they lack demand, but because demand outruns discipline.

In private practice, volume is seductive. Full clinics and packed OR days feel like progress. But volume without margin accelerates exhaustion. Every additional patient brings not just revenue, but cost—staff time, administrative burden, denial risk, emotional labor.

Margin, not motion, is what sustains a practice.

This is why experienced private practitioners become obsessed with overhead—not as an accounting exercise, but as a survival instinct. Staffing ratios, payer mix, revenue cycle, collections discipline, pricing strategy, and physical footprint quietly determine whether effort compounds or evaporates.

Private practice punishes the belief that hard work alone is enough.

Why Private Practices Rarely Collapse—They Erode

Private practices almost never fail dramatically.

They erode quietly.

A staffing hire justified as temporary becomes permanent. Overhead inches upward while reimbursement inches downward. Small inefficiencies are tolerated because confronting them feels uncomfortable. Financial data is reviewed less frequently because it's unpleasant. Partners stop having hard conversations because things are "mostly fine."

Private practice does not forgive avoidance. What institutions buffer through scale, private practices surface personally.

The danger is not a bad year. The danger is a slow drift away from coherence.

The Financial Reality of Private Practice

One of the great misunderstandings about private practice is that physicians step into it fully formed—as owners, decision-makers, and beneficiaries of the economics from day one.

That is rarely how it works.

Most young physicians enter private practice as employees first, even when the practice is physician-owned. They are paid a salary, sometimes with productivity incentives, and are insulated—temporarily—from the true financial mechanics of the business. Overhead is abstract. Collections are someone else's problem. Facility costs, staffing ratios, payer mix, and capital expenditures exist in the background.

This phase is intentional. It allows the physician to build clinical confidence, referral relationships, and volume without simultaneously carrying business risk. But it also creates a delayed reckoning.

After a few years—often two to five—the conversation shifts. Partnership is offered. Equity is discussed. Buy-ins are calculated. Suddenly, the physician is no longer just producing revenue; they are responsible for how that revenue is generated, captured, and retained.

This transition is where many private practice careers are made—or quietly derailed.

Partnership does not simply increase income. It changes incentives. As an employee, inefficiency is frustrating. As a partner, inefficiency is expensive. Decisions that once felt administrative—how many staff to hire, how to schedule clinic, which payers to accept—become existential.

Private practice asks a hard question at this stage: *Do you want ownership, or do you want insulation?* The answer is not obvious, and there is no shame in choosing either. But the consequences differ.

Where Private Practice Actually Makes Money

Private practice profitability is not primarily driven by professional fees alone. In fact, professional fees are often the least scalable component of the business.

The real leverage comes from capturing care that would otherwise be outsourced.

In-office procedures are a clear example. When procedures that are safe, efficient, and appropriate for the office setting are moved out of the operating room, the economics shift dramatically. The practice retains facility fees, controls scheduling, reduces cancellations, and compresses time between evaluation and treatment. The patient experience often improves. The margin widens.

Similarly, facility fees—whether through office-based procedure suites or ambulatory surgery centers—can transform a practice's financial profile. When structured correctly, these fees reward efficiency and volume without proportionally increasing overhead. When structured poorly, they become capital-intensive liabilities.

The difference lies in discipline and utilization.

Ancillary services represent another inflection point.

In-house audiology and hearing aid dispensing are among the most powerful—and misunderstood—financial engines in otolaryngology. When audiology is integrated thoughtfully, it improves continuity of care, reduces leakage, and creates a recurring revenue stream that is not tied directly to physician hours. Hearing aids, in particular, can be highly lucrative when patient trust is strong and counseling is done well.

This is not "selling." It is care consolidation. The patient benefits from fewer handoffs. The practice benefits from margin stability.

In-office CT scanning follows a similar logic. When imaging is brought in-house, practices gain speed, diagnostic control, and capture revenue that would otherwise leave the ecosystem. The key, again, is utilization. A CT scanner that is used well becomes an asset. One that is underutilized becomes a drag on cash flow.

Private practice rewards physicians who think in terms of systems, not transactions.

The Psychological Shift of Ownership

What makes these financial mechanisms powerful is not just the money—they change how physicians think.

Ownership sharpens attention. Physicians who become partners begin to notice patterns they previously ignored: no-show rates, cancellation trends, payer behavior, staff turnover, and the true cost of "just one more hire." Time becomes financial. Efficiency becomes personal.

This shift can be invigorating or unsettling.

Some physicians find deep satisfaction in this clarity. They enjoy understanding the full machine and optimizing it. Others realize they preferred the predictability of employment and the distance it provided from these concerns.

Neither response is wrong. But private practice does not allow ambiguity for long.

The Risk Beneath the Reward

The same mechanisms that create upside in private practice also create exposure.

Ancillaries require upfront capital. Facility ownership concentrates risk. Audiology programs depend on staff stability and ethical discipline. Imaging equipment depreciates regardless of volume. Partnership means shared fate—good and bad.

This is why private practice is not merely a financial decision. It is a temperament test.

Physicians who tolerate uncertainty, engage with numbers honestly, and address problems early tend to thrive. Those who avoid financial reality or defer uncomfortable decisions often struggle, even in otherwise successful practices.

Private practice does not forgive denial.

What This Means for the Young Physician

For early-career physicians, the takeaway is not that private practice is superior or inferior. It is that private practice is different.

Entering as an employee is not a failure. It is often the right move. But partnership should be approached with eyes open—not as a reward, but as a redefinition of responsibility.

Understanding where money is made, where it leaks, and how ancillaries and facilities alter the equation is not optional if ownership is your goal. Financial literacy is not greed in private practice; it is stewardship.

Private practice gives you the chance to align care, culture, and compensation in a way few other models allow. But it demands that you understand the machine you are stepping into.

Freedom, in private practice, is not given.

It is earned—through clarity, discipline, and responsibility.

Concierge Medicine

11

Concierge medicine is often misunderstood because people argue about it as if it were one thing.

It is not.

Sometimes concierge is a retainer model layered on top of insurance. Sometimes it's direct care. Sometimes it's a boutique version of a conventional practice with better access and more time. Sometimes it's a hybrid where patients pay for the visit but still use insurance for surgery and facility fees.

But beneath those variations, concierge medicine has one defining feature: it renegotiates the physician–patient contract.

It changes what is being purchased. It changes expectations. And it changes where accountability sits.

If you do not understand that new contract, concierge medicine can feel either like salvation or betrayal. In reality, it's neither. It's a different operating system.

Why Concierge Medicine Exists

Concierge medicine did not emerge because physicians suddenly became less altruistic. It emerged because the traditional contract between physicians and the healthcare system became increasingly misaligned.

F. Sokoya, *Building Your Otolaryngology Practice*,
https://doi.org/10.1007/978-3-032-27397-0_11

In the insurance-driven model, physicians are asked to deliver relational, judgment-intensive care inside workflows designed for throughput. Time fragments. Access becomes a KPI rather than a clinical value. Administrative burden crowds out presence. The physician's attention becomes the scarce resource—rationed into short appointments and filtered through processes that often do not reflect what the patient actually needed.

Dr. Ashley Agan described the inflection point in plain language. She wasn't leaving medicine; she was leaving a pace that felt incompatible with good care:

> The squeeze to see more patients, faster… was becoming untenable. I just thought, *this is not the way I want to practice medicine.*

Concierge medicine is a response to that tension. It tries to restore what many patients and physicians quietly miss: continuity, responsiveness, and time.

The deeper question is not whether this is understandable. It's whether it is sustainable and ethically coherent.

The New Contract: Access for Commitment

At its core, concierge medicine replaces third-party opacity with direct alignment.

Patients pay for access—shorter waits, longer visits, direct communication, and the sense that their physician actually knows them. In exchange, the physician commits to a smaller panel and deeper longitudinal responsibility.

This is not theory. It's measurable.

A national survey of retainer ("concierge") practices found that physicians in retainer models reported dramatically smaller panel sizes than non-retainer counterparts (mean ~898 vs. ~2303) [1], saw fewer patients per day, and were more likely to offer features like enhanced coordination and around-the-clock access [2]. Concierge medicine changes the denominator. It buys time by reducing volume.

Agan's practice describes what this looks like operationally in ENT. She schedules a full hour for new patients and commonly 30 minutes for follow-ups, which allows the encounter to feel human rather than rushed. She also emphasized the practical difference it makes for physicians:

"All my notes get done by the end of the day. There's nothing hovering over me after clinic."

Concierge medicine does not just change how patients experience care. It changes how physicians experience their own work.

The Concierge Patient Is Not Who You Think

One of the most common misconceptions about concierge medicine is that it is simply medicine for rich people.

Agan expected this too—and found it wasn't true in the way people imagine:

> When I first got into it, there was a part of me that was like, 'Am I only going to be taking care of rich people?' … It's not like that at all.

Instead, she found that the concierge patient is often defined less by wealth than by values and structure. Many of her patients live outside the typical insurance model or engage it differently: small business owners who self-budget for emergencies, families in Christian health-sharing arrangements who demand price transparency, and patients with high-deductible plans who realize they are paying out-of-pocket regardless.

As she put it:

> It's more about what people value than what's in their bank account.

That distinction matters because it reframes concierge medicine as a market segmentation around time, transparency, and control—not simply income.

It also aligns with what the research suggests: concierge and retainer practices tend to serve fewer Medicaid patients and fewer underserved populations [2]. This does not automatically condemn the model, but it makes the ethical trade-off impossible to ignore. Concierge expands access for some by narrowing access for others.

That is the contract.

What We Know—And What We Do not—About Outcomes

Many people assume concierge medicine must improve outcomes because it increases time and continuity. That might be true in certain contexts. But the literature is more cautious.

A 2024 review of concierge medicine studies found that concierge care is generally associated with higher patient satisfaction and engagement, and may increase preventive care utilization, but evidence on hard outcomes and system-wide costs remains mixed and limited by study design [3].

That matters because concierge medicine is often marketed as "better medicine." The honest version is: it is often a better experience, often clearer communication and coordination, and potentially better preventive alignment—but outcomes are still context dependent.

The real question is not "Is concierge medicine better?" It's "Better for whom, under what conditions, and at what cost?"

ENT Concierge Economics: The Part Most People Miss

Concierge medicine is often discussed through the lens of primary care membership models. ENT is different.

Much of ENT is episodic, procedure-driven, and event-based. That changes the economics.

Agan explained something most physicians overlook: for many ENT surgeries, even in a concierge model, patients still use insurance for the facility and anesthesia while paying the surgeon fee directly. When patients learn where the costs actually sit, the psychology changes:

> Once people realize the surgeon fee isn't the biggest fee in that bundle, everyone's like, 'Oh—that's not that bad.'

She also highlighted an operational lever that can make concierge ENT not only viable but also competitive: facility selection and bundling. She described patients with high deductibles being quoted staggering hospital prices for routine pediatric procedures—and then choosing her practice because a surgery center bundled anesthesia and facility fees at a far lower total cost.

Concierge medicine, in this form, is not always more expensive. Sometimes it's more transparent. Sometimes it's simply more rational.

Another underappreciated advantage is cash flow. Concierge and cash-pay models often eliminate the long, messy accounts receivable cycles of insurance billing. Agan described it plainly: patients pay at the visit, and surgical fees are paid predictably in advance. The practice becomes easier to forecast and less vulnerable to administrative denial friction.

This is what people mean when they say concierge "simplifies" practice. Not that it becomes easy, but that the financial mechanics become legible.

Membership Versus Fee-for-Service: Why ENT Is Different

Most concierge discourse assumes a membership model because primary care is longitudinal.

ENT often is not.

Agan tested membership early and found the reality quickly:

> Maybe one or two people opted for membership… it didn't translate.

Her explanation is simple and important: most ENT patients come for a specific problem, get it addressed, and move on. That does not mean there's no continuity—family referrals and recurrent conditions absolutely exist—but the engine of ENT is not the same as primary care.

This is why concierge ENT may fit better as fee-for-service rather than pure membership. Trying to force a primary-care membership model onto an episodic specialty often creates the wrong incentives and the wrong expectations.

Operational Reality: Boundaries Are the Whole Game

From the outside, concierge medicine looks like fewer patients, more time, and predictable revenue.

But psychologically and operationally, it can be demanding if boundaries are not designed carefully.

When patients pay directly, expectations sharpen. Availability becomes part of the product. If boundaries are vague, your life becomes porous—texts, calls, and small questions expanding into constant cognitive load.

What makes Agan's story particularly valuable is that it's realistic. She provides meaningful access without being consumed by it:

> My surgery patients have my cell phone… but they really don't bother me outside of hours.

This is a reminder that boundaries are not just policies. They are culture. When expectations are clear and the experience is high-quality, many patients become more respectful, not more demanding.

Concierge medicine succeeds or fails on boundary design—response-time expectations, communication channels, after-hours policies, and clarity around what is included versus billed separately. Without that structure, concierge becomes what it claims to solve: endless access pressure.

Ethics and the Weight of the Model

Concierge medicine forces medicine's ethical tension into the open: the tension between equity and efficiency, between individual experience and population access.

Economists studying concierge-like arrangements find stronger evidence of selection based on income than on health status—meaning these models segment patients primarily by ability to pay [4]. The American College of Physicians has also acknowledged that while concierge/direct primary care models may improve access and continuity for some, they raise concerns about reduced access for those unable to pay and potential contribution to primary care shortages [5].

This does not mean concierge medicine is unethical by definition. It means it carries ethical weight. If you adopt it, you should do so with eyes open and language honest.

Concierge medicine is not an escape hatch. It is a choice about who you serve and how you define obligation.

Concierge Medicine as a Phase, Not an Identity

One of the most practical reframes is this: concierge medicine does not have to be permanent.

For some physicians, it is a late-career model that preserves energy and meaning. For others, it is a mid-career recalibration after years of throughput-driven practice. For a few, it becomes a lifelong identity.

Agan's advice to young physicians was candid and important:

> It's the harder road. It's going to take longer to get busy.

But she also framed the long-term appeal clearly: less exposure to payer rules, less administrative overhead, and a business model that feels like a straighter line.

Concierge should not be entered as a resentful reaction to a broken system. Resentment creates sloppy boundaries. Sloppy boundaries destroy concierge practices.

It should be chosen as a positive model—grounded in self-knowledge and clarity about what kind of work you want to do.

The Deeper Question

Concierge medicine ultimately forces a question that extends beyond economics:

What do you owe your patients—and what do you owe your own life?

Traditional models hide this question inside bureaucracy and volume. Concierge models bring it to the surface. That clarity can be liberating. It can also be heavy.

Concierge medicine is not about abandoning medicine's ideals. It is about choosing which ideals you are best equipped to serve—and doing so without illusion.

Concierge medicine is a renegotiated physician–patient contract, not just a pricing model.

It reliably reduces panel size and increases access features, but may alter the patient mix served [2].

Evidence suggests improved satisfaction and engagement, while outcomes and cost effects remain mixed [3].

Equity concerns are real and largely driven by income-based selection [4, 5].

ENT concierge often functions best as fee-for-service rather than membership, reflecting episodic demand.

Concierge success depends less on branding than on boundary design and expectation management.

Bibliography

1. Raffoul M, Moore M, Kamerow D, Bazemore A. A primary care panel size of 2500 is neither accurate nor reasonable. J Am Board Fam Med. 2016.
2. Alexander GC, Kurlander J, Wynia MK. Physicians in retainer ("concierge") practice: a national survey of physician, patient, and practice characteristics. J Gen Intern Med. 2005;
3. Alhawshani S, et al. A literature review on the impact of concierge medicine services on individual healthcare. J Family Med Prim Care. 2024.
4. Leive A, et al. On resource allocation in health care: the case of concierge medicine Int J Ind Organ. 2023.
5. Doherty R. Assessing the patient care implications of "concierge" and direct primary care. Ann Intern Med (ACP Policy Paper). 2015.

12 Lessons from the Field

After you strip away titles, contracts, and practice models, something surprising remains.

The physicians who thrive do not share the same jobs. They do not work in the same settings. They do not even define success the same way. What they share is not a structure—it is a set of behaviors and decisions that repeat across environments.

This chapter is not about which path to choose. It is about recognizing the patterns that endure regardless of path—and the mistakes that quietly undermine otherwise brilliant careers.

What Successful Physicians Do Consistently

Across every interview, across every model—academic, hospital-employed, private practice, concierge—certain behaviors surfaced again and again.

Successful physicians understand incentives before they judge systems. They don't romanticize or demonize environments; they learn how those environments actually work. They see metrics not as moral judgments, but as signals. That fluency allows them to operate without constant friction.

They take ownership early—even when they are not owners. This was especially clear in Jon Young's experience inside a large multispecialty system. Despite being "shielded" from overhead

F. Sokoya, *Building Your Otolaryngology Practice*,
https://doi.org/10.1007/978-3-032-27397-0_12

and billing, he behaved as if the practice were his: building subspecialty services, expanding scope, advocating for resources, and pushing the system to support growth rather than passively accepting constraints. The mindset came first; the authority followed.

They build leverage before they need it. Ducic did this through outcomes and intellectual rigor. Winkler did it by building a division before it officially existed. Henriquez did it by becoming indispensable clinically and educationally before transitioning settings. Barham did it by mastering the economics before scaling. None of them waited for leverage to be granted.

And they invest deeply in relationships—often quietly. Referring physicians, staff, administrators, partners. These relationships outlast job titles. Jon Young emphasized this in a subtle way: his success in expanding pediatric ENT services came not from formal authority, but from being the person others trusted to handle complexity when no one else wanted it.

The pattern is clear: successful physicians behave like stewards long before they are treated like leaders.

The Most Common Mistakes (and Why Smart People Make Them)

Just as striking as the success patterns were the failure patterns.

The most common mistake was chasing the wrong signal. Early-career physicians often optimize for salary, RVUs, or prestige, assuming alignment will follow. It rarely does. When incentives don't match values, dissatisfaction grows quietly.

Another recurring mistake was delaying financial and operational literacy. Many physicians assumed they would "learn the business later." By the time they did, leverage had already shifted. Barham's observation that overhead matters more than revenue came not from theory, but from watching smart people bleed margin while celebrating growth.

Avoidance was another theme. Avoidance of conflict with partners. Avoidance of uncomfortable conversations with leadership.

Avoidance of numbers. Private practice punishes this immediately. Hospital systems punish it slowly—but just as decisively.

Finally, over-specialization too early appeared repeatedly. Jon Young spoke candidly about the danger of narrowing scope before understanding the ecosystem. In his practice, breadth—pediatric airway, craniofacial work, multidisciplinary care—created durability. Narrowing prematurely often reduced optionality rather than increasing it.

These mistakes are not due to incompetence. They arise because medicine trains physicians to delay self-interest, defer authority, and trust systems. Those habits serve patients well. They serve careers poorly if left unexamined.

How Careers Actually Evolve

No one's career followed the path they were taught in training.

Academic practice was often a foundation, not a destination. Private practice was often an evolution, not a rebellion. Leadership roles emerged organically from problem-solving, not ambition. Financial success became about optionality, not validation.

Henriquez's arc illustrates this clearly. Years at Grady, teaching Emory residents, publishing, advancing facial trauma and skull base work—this was not a detour. It was preparation. When he transitioned into a community-based practice, he carried academic rigor with him, but gained flexibility and fulfillment the institution could no longer provide.

Jon Young's experience reinforced another truth: careers bend toward where effort meets opportunity. His growth within a large system came from identifying unmet needs and filling them relentlessly—not from waiting for permission.

The lesson is uncomfortable but liberating: careers are authored, not inherited.

Redefining Success over Time

Success is not static.

Early in a career, success often looks like selection: getting the job, building volume, proving competence. Mid-career, it shifts toward alignment: autonomy, leverage, sustainability. Later, success becomes about impact: mentoring others, shaping systems, leaving something that persists.

Winkler's emphasis on mentorship and fellowship training reflected this shift. Ducic's influence—measured not by title, but by the surgeons he trained and the standards he set—embodied it. Barham's clarity around economics and structure demonstrated that fulfillment often comes from coherence rather than chaos.

Jon Young offered a quieter version of this insight. For him, success became less about proving expertise and more about building programs that worked—systems that could sustain good care without constant heroics.

The definition changes. Ignoring that evolution is how people burn out.

Across interviews, one diagnostic question emerged—often implicitly:

Does my environment amplify my best work—or extract from it?

In academia, this question reveals whether the institution is a platform or a constraint.

In hospital employment, it distinguishes support from surveillance.

In private practice, it separates ownership from burden.

In concierge medicine, it clarifies whether intimacy is energizing or draining.

Physicians who thrive revisit this question regularly. Those who don't often wake up years later wondering when dissatisfaction became permanent.

Medicine is a long game.

No practice model is permanent. No decision is final. Identity should never be outsourced to an institution, a contract, or a title.

The physicians whose careers endure are not purists. They adapt. They learn. They course-correct. They treat clarity as a skill and self-awareness as a responsibility.

The most dangerous assumption in medicine is that someone else is steering.

The most durable careers are those that are consciously authored, one decision at a time.

13 Adapting to the Future of Healthcare: Without Losing Yourself

Most conversations about the future of healthcare are noisy and shallow.

They fixate on tools—artificial intelligence, telemedicine, automation, value-based care—while missing the deeper truth: tools change faster than incentives. If you understand the incentives, the future becomes less frightening and more navigable.

Physicians are rarely good futurists. We are, however, excellent pattern recognizers. We spend our lives identifying signals amid noise, distinguishing what matters from what doesn't, and making decisions under uncertainty.

The future of medicine doesn't require prediction. It requires clarity.

The Mistake Everyone Makes About the Future

The most common error physicians make when thinking about the future is assuming that it will arrive as a clean break—one day medicine looks like this, the next day it looks like something else.

That's not how change happens.

Change in healthcare is almost always additive and asymmetric. New forces pile on top of old ones. Measurement expands without replacing judgment. Technology accelerates certain tasks while exposing weaknesses in others. Capital consolidates slowly, then suddenly.

F. Sokoya, *Building Your Otolaryngology Practice*,
https://doi.org/10.1007/978-3-032-27397-0_13

The danger is not change itself.

The danger is anchoring your identity to a structure that no longer protects you.

The Forces That Are Actually Reshaping Medicine

The future of healthcare is being shaped less by innovation than by pressure.

Consolidation continues because scale confers negotiating power. Measurement creeps outward because systems need proxies for performance. Capital replaces hierarchy because money moves faster than committees. Technology compresses time and distance because inefficiency is no longer tolerated. Patients expect access, transparency, and responsiveness because those expectations have been set everywhere else in their lives.

None of these forces are ideological. They are structural.

Arguing with them is like arguing with gravity.

The physicians who struggle are often those who mistake resistance for integrity. The physicians who adapt do something quieter: they learn how the system works without allowing it to define who they are.

What Will Become Commoditized

Commoditization is not a moral judgment. It is an economic one.

In the years ahead, anything that is routine, repeatable, and easily standardized will move toward lower margins and lower differentiation. This includes routine visits, standardized procedures, pattern-recognition tasks, and care models built purely on availability.

Competence will remain necessary—but it will be table stakes.

Physicians whose primary value is "being there" will find themselves increasingly replaceable. Systems will optimize around them. Technology will assist, then automate portions of their work. Payment will follow.

This is not pessimism. It is the predictable outcome of scale.

What Will Not Be Commoditized

What resists commoditization is not knowledge—it is judgment.

Judgment under uncertainty. Managing edge cases. Integrating conflicting information. Navigating ambiguity when there is no algorithm. Building trust over time. Teaching others how to think, not just what to do.

Leadership, synthesis, and systems design will matter more, not less.

This is why the earlier chapters emphasized research, ownership, and old-school medicine. These are not nostalgic ideas. They are defensive skills against commoditization.

The future will reward physicians who can *see*, not just execute.

Artificial Intelligence: The Wrong Fear and the Right One

The wrong fear is that AI will replace physicians.

That fear misunderstands what AI actually does.

AI does not replace judgment. It exposes its absence.

Pattern recognition will improve. Documentation will accelerate. Diagnostic assistance will become ubiquitous. But the physician who relies on these tools without understanding their limits will be more vulnerable, not less.

AI rewards clarity of thought. It punishes shallow practice.

For physicians who know what they're doing, AI will be a force multiplier—freeing time, reducing friction, and expanding reach. For those who don't, it will reveal gaps they could previously hide behind volume or busyness.

The future does not belong to those who memorize more facts.

It belongs to those who integrate information into coherent decisions. AI may help you navigate the NCCN guidelines, but it cannot account for the socioeconomic realities and psychosocial nuances that determine which treatment a patient will realistically follow.

The Adaptive Physician

Across every model—academic, employed, private, concierge—the physicians most likely to thrive in the future share a recognizable profile.

They are model-agnostic. They don't define themselves by where they work, but by how they work. They understand finances well enough to avoid dependence. They are comfortable reinventing parts of their practice without reinventing their values.

They are not emotionally attached to structures. They can leave, build, or change without identity collapse. They don't wait for permission to grow. They don't outsource authorship of their careers.

Most importantly, they remain students of the system—curious about incentives, skeptical of metrics, and disciplined about alignment.

The Trap of Nostalgia

Nostalgia is the quiet enemy of adaptation.

There was never a golden age of medicine without constraint. There was only a period when constraints were different and less visible. Longing for a past that cannot return makes physicians brittle. It encourages purity tests instead of practical solutions.

The future does not punish ignorance as harshly as it punishes rigidity.

Adaptation is not betrayal.

It is how agency is preserved.

The One Skill That Matters Most

The future of healthcare does not belong to the smartest physicians, the busiest physicians, or the most credentialed physicians.

It belongs to those who can see clearly, adapt deliberately, and refuse to outsource ownership of their professional lives.

The future will keep changing.
The incentives will keep shifting.
The structures will keep evolving.

What endures is your ability to recognize what matters—and to move toward it intentionally.

That is not prediction.
That is preparation.

14 Your Personalized Action Plan

By now, you have seen the landscape clearly.

You've examined the structures that shape modern medical careers—academia, hospital employment, private practice, concierge models—not as ideologies, but as systems with incentives, constraints, and trade-offs. You've seen how careers actually unfold, how leverage is built, how misalignment erodes satisfaction, and how adaptation preserves agency.

What remains is not more knowledge.

It is translation.

This final chapter is not about telling you what to do. It is about helping you decide what to do next, in a way that is coherent with who you are and where you are in your career.

Start Where You Are, Not Where You Think You Should Be

The most common mistake physicians make at this stage is trying to design an ideal future without honestly assessing the present.

Before making plans, ask a simpler question: *What phase am I actually in?*

Early career often centers on competence, confidence, and credibility. Mid-career shifts toward autonomy, leverage, and sustainability. Later career asks about impact, legacy, and stewardship. These phases overlap, but they are not interchangeable.

F. Sokoya, *Building Your Otolaryngology Practice*,
https://doi.org/10.1007/978-3-032-27397-0_14

Trying to optimize for autonomy before competence is fragile.
Trying to chase validation after clarity is corrosive.
An honest action plan begins with self-location.

Audit Your Environment

Every practice environment either amplifies your best work or extracts from it.

This is not about comfort. It's about signal.

Pay attention to these four things:

1. Where your energy goes.
2. What work feels generative versus draining.
3. Which constraints feel tolerable and which feel suffocating.
4. Whether growth feels possible or merely rhetorical.

If your environment consistently rewards the parts of you you value most, small frustrations are survivable. If it consistently extracts from those parts, no amount of compensation or prestige will compensate long term.

This is the quiet diagnostic most satisfied physicians revisit repeatedly.

Build Leverage Before You Need It

Leverage is not something you negotiate for in a crisis.

It is something you accumulate when things are stable.

That leverage may come from:

- Skills that are difficult to replace.
- Relationships that outlast roles.
- Financial literacy that reduces dependence.
- Reputation for reliability and judgment.
- Optionality—the credible ability to say no.

You do not need all of these. But you need enough that your career does not feel trapped.

An action plan that does not include leverage is not a plan. It is hope!

Choose What You Will Learn Next

Medicine rewards continuous learning—but not indiscriminately.

At every stage, ask yourself: *What knowledge would most expand my agency right now?*

Early on, that may be clinical mastery.

Later, it may be finance, operations, leadership, or negotiation.

At another point, it may be teaching, research, or systems design.

Learning should be strategic, not reflexive.

The physicians who thrive long term are not those who know the most things. They are those who learn the *right* things at the *right* time.

Learn like your career (and life) depends on it.

Design Constraints, Don't Just Escape Them

Many career moves are framed as escapes: leaving academia, leaving hospital employment, leaving volume, leaving bureaucracy.

Escape is rarely durable.

Sustainable careers are built by designing constraints, not avoiding them. Every model has friction. The question is which friction you are willing to manage.

An effective action plan doesn't ask, *How do I get rid of constraints?*

It asks, *Which constraints am I willing to live with—and which am I not?*

That clarity prevents regret.

Revisit the Question That Matters

Across all the interviews, all the models, all the paths, one question kept resurfacing:

Does my current trajectory move me closer to the physician I want to be—or further away from them?

Not the job title.
Not the compensation.
Not the external validation.
The physician.

Careers drift when this question goes unasked. They stabilize when it is revisited regularly, without drama.

Your Plan Should Be Alive

A final warning.

The worst action plans are static. They lock you into assumptions that will change. Medicine will change. You will change. Your priorities will shift.

Your action plan should be alive—reviewed annually, adjusted deliberately, and never treated as a verdict.

Adaptation is not failure.
Course correction is not weakness.
Reinvention is not betrayal.

There is no perfect model.
There is no final arrival.
There is only alignment—temporary, revisitable, earned.
The goal of this book was never to tell you where to go.
It was to help you see clearly enough to choose well. If you can do that—again and again—your career will not be perfect.

But it will be yours.

The most durable medical careers are not inherited.

They are *authored*—one clear decision at a time. And authors, by definition, can revise.

Index

A
Academic medicine, 8, 9
Academic practice, 87
  clinical cases, 51
    Ducic, Yadro, 52–53
    Henriquez, Oswaldo, 56–57
    Winkler, Andrew, 54, 55
  compensation, 58
  compression, 58
  credibility, 53
  gravity of, 58
  institutional alignment, 60
  leadership, 57, 59
  misalignment, 60
  optimization, 52
  persistent misalignment, 57
  research and innovation, 59
  ripple effect of mentorship, 59
  structural ceiling, 58
  teaching, 59
  tertiary-and quaternary care, 53
  thriving vs. burning out, 52
Access, 30
Action, 2
Action plan, 98–100
Adaptive physician, 94
Agency, 18
AI-based ambient transcription tools, 32
Alignment, 2–3
Ancillary services, 72, 73
Artificial intelligence (AI), 93–94
  transcription, 32
Assumption, dangerous in medicine, 89
Audiology, 72, 73
Autonomy, 55
Avoidance, as career risk, 86

B
Burnout, 34

C
Career decisions, 2
Career durability, 40, 89
Career path in otolaryngology, 4
Career planning, 97
Careers drift, 100
Careers evolution, physicians, 87
Cash pay, 26, 27
Clinic templates, 30
Clinical research
  as meaning infrastructure, 35–36
  leverage inside system, 36–37
  productive, 38
Collections, 26
Committees, 18, 21
Commoditization, 92, 93

F. Sokoya, *Building Your Otolaryngology Practice*,
https://doi.org/10.1007/978-3-032-27397-0

Communication, 19, 76, 77
Compensation, 46, 47, 58
Competence, 2–3, 92, 97, 98
Compression, 58
Concierge medicine
  access for communication, 76, 77
  advantages, 81
  challenges, 81
  defining feature, 75
  direct care, 75
  ENT economics, 78, 79
  ethics and the weight of the model, 81
  ideals, medical practice, 82
  membership versus fee-for-service, 79–80
  mid-career recalibration, 81
  misconceptions, 77
  operational reality, 80
  outcomes, 78
  panel size, 82
  retainer practices, 76
  time fragments, 76
  traditional healthcare system, 75
Confidence, 97
Consolidation, 92
Continuity of standards, 55
Core professional competency, 24
Corporate trade-off, 65–66
Cosmetic surgery, 54
Credibility, 97

D
Design constraints, 99
Diagnostic question, career, 88
Diffusion-of-innovations, 38
Direct care, 75

E
Early-career physicians, 44
Early career rewards, 4
EHR log analyses, 31
Eudaimonia, 3

F
Facial plastic surgery, 54
Fee-for-service, 80
Fellowship training, 88
Financial foundations
  cash pay and aesthetics, 26–27
  collections, 26
  financial literacy, 24
  overhead, 27
  practical definition, 28
  private equity, 28
  quick reality check, 24–25
  revenue, 25
  two financial realities, 25
  wRVUs, 26
Financial literacy, 24, 74
Financial reality, 71–72
Future of medicine
  artificial intelligence, 93–94
  change in healthcare, 91, 95
  commoditization, 92, 93
  nostalgia, 94
  physician adaptation, 91, 92, 94
  physicians, 95
  professional identity, 92
  professional ownership, 95
  structural forces, 92

G
Gathering information process, 49, 50
Goal setting, 100
Goodhart's law, 62–64

H
HCAHPS surveys, 63
Healthcare economics, 24
Hearing aids, 72
Hidden tax on productivity, 31, 32
High-functioning systems, 67
Hospital-employed practice
  corporate trade-off, 65–66
  Goodhart's law, 62–64

HCAHPS surveys, 63
high-functioning systems, 67
language changes, 62
leverage, 64
metrics, 67
net promoter score, 63
paradox of, 66
practical autonomy, 65
relationships, 67
signals, 62
system, as platform, 64
Hospital employment, 9, 10
Hospital incentives, 62

I
Incentive alignment, 14
Incentives shape identity, 14, 15
Information asymmetry, 49
Innovation
as differentiation, 38–39
long view, 40
teaching multiplies impact, 39–40
In-office procedures, 72
Intellectual authority, 53
Intellectual capital, 36
Intentionality, program design, 54

L
Late-career model, 81
Late career rewards, 4
Leadership, 21
changes, 57
supportive, 55
Learning, 99
Leverage, 97–99
Leverage inside system, 36–37
Lived experience, 87
Long view, 40
Low-value services, 27

M
Major academic center, 53
Masked model, 10, 11
Meaning infrastructure, 35–36
Medical group, 62
Mentorship, 88
Metrics, 21, 33, 34
Microvascular free tissue transfer, 52
Mid-career recalibration, 81
Mid-career rewards, 4
Mistakes, common in physician careers, 86

N
National Academies' Learning Health System framework, 37
Negotiating contracts
calibrated questions, 48
call, 46
compensation structures, 46, 47
early-career physicians, 44
gathering information process, 49, 50
leverage, 44, 45
malpractice insurance, 47
non-compete, 46
RVU, 46
salary, 46
tail coverage, 47
walking away, 48, 49
Net promoter score, 63
Non-compete, 46

O
Operant conditioning, 14
Optionality, 22
OR time, 32, 33
Overhead, 27
Over-specialization, 87
Ownership, physicians, 55

P
Pajama time, 31
Payer mix, 26
Periodic reflection, 4
Physician adaptation, 94
Physician agency, 99
Physician autonomy, 11
Physician behavior, 22
Physician contract negotiations, 43
Physician employment, 8
Physician interviews, 85
Physician–patient contract, 75
Practice building, 17, 28
Practice environment, 98
Practice landscape
  academic medicine, 8, 9
  hospital employment, 9, 10
  incentives shape identity, 14, 15
  masked model, 10, 11
  private equity, 12, 13
  private practice, 11, 12
  structural shift, 7–8
Practice model, 5, 88
Price of ownership, 11
Primary care membership
    models, 78
Private equity, 12, 13, 28
Private practice, 7, 11, 12, 87, 88
  audiology, 72
  avoidance, 74
  in discipline and utilization, 72
  facility fees, 72
  financial reality, 71–72
  hearing aids, 72
  in-office procedures, 72, 73
  physicians, 74
  professional fees, 72
  profitability, 72
  psychological shift
    of ownership, 73
  redefinition of responsibility, 74
  risk, 73
Productive research, 37, 38
Productivity optimization
  access, 30
  AI transcription, 32
  burnout, 34
  clinic templates, 30
  documentation, 31–32
  hidden tax on productivity, 31, 32
  metrics, 33, 34
  OR time, 32, 33
  pajama time, 31
  sustainability, 34
  time, 29
Professional identity, 1, 92
Professional reputation, 19
Psychological shift of ownership, 73
Publications, 38

Q
Quick reality check, 24–25

R
Referral relationships, 19
Relative value units (RVUs), 46
Retainer ("concierge")
    practices, 76

S
Scholarly output, 36
Self assessment, 99
Self-knowledge, 1, 5, 6
Shaping modern reconstructive
    paradigms, 53
Social media, 20, 21
SQUIRE 2.0 guidelines, 37
Stoicism, principles, 17
Strategic decision-making, 99
Structural forces, 92
Structural shift, 7–8
Success, 3
Success, redefined over time, 88
Sustainability, 34
Systems design, as sucess, 88

T
Tail coverage, 47
Teaching multiplies impact, 39–40
Three A's, 20

Throughput-driven practice, 81
Time, as currency, 18
Time fragments, 76
Time-motion studies, 31
Traditional healthcare system, 75

U
University hospitals, 52

V
Values, 3–6, 58
Voss's approach, 43
Voss's framework, 43

W
Work relative value units (wRVUs), 23, 25, 26

GPSR Compliance

The European Union's (EU) General Product Safety Regulation (GPSR) is a set of rules that requires consumer products to be safe and our obligations to ensure this.

If you have any concerns about our products, you can contact us on ProductSafety@springernature.com

In case Publisher is established outside the EU, the EU authorized representative is:

Springer Nature Customer Service Center GmbH
Europaplatz 3
69115 Heidelberg, Germany

Batch number: 10726064

Printed by Printforce, the Netherlands